KW-147-628

JOHN STUART BARKER

Auscultation of the Heart

WITH NOTES ON OBSERVATION AND PALPATION

Richard W. D. Turner

OBE, MA, MD, FRCP, FRCP(Edin)
Formerly Reader in Medicine, University of Edinburgh,
Edinburgh, UK

Ronald G. Gold

MB BS, FRCP, FRACP
Clinical Lecturer in Cardiology, University of Newcastle upon Tyne;
Consultant Cardiologist, Regional Cardiothoracic Centre, Freeman Hospital,
Newcastle upon Tyne, UK

FIFTH EDITION

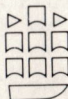

CHURCHILL LIVINGSTONE
EDINBURGH LONDON MELBOURNE AND NEW YORK 1984

CHURCHILL LIVINGSTONE
Medical Division of Longman Group Limited

Distributed in the United States of America by
Churchill Livingstone Inc., 1560 Broadway, New York,
N. Y. 10036, and by associated companies, branches
and representatives throughout the world.

First Edition 1963
Second Edition 1964
Third Edition 1968
Fourth Edition 1972
Fifth Edition 1984

ISBN 0 443 02886 9

British Library Cataloguing in Publication Data
Turner, Richard W.D.
    Auscultation of the heart. — 5th ed.
    I. Title   II. Gold, Ronald G.
    616.1′20754   RC683.5.A9

Library of Congress Cataloging in Publication Data
Turner, Richard W. D. (Richard Wainwright Duke)
    Auscultation of the heart.

    Includes index.
    1. Auscultation.   2. Heart — Diseases — Diagnosis.
3. Palpation.   I. Gold, Ronald G. (Ronald Geoffrey)
II. Title   [DNLM: 1. Heart Auscultation.   WG 141.5.A9
T951a]
RC683.5.A9T87   1984   616.1′20754   84-4931

Printed in Singapore by The Print House (Pte) Ltd

Preface to Fifth Edition

Twelve years have passed since the publication of the Fourth Edition of this book and there have been a number of important changes in the field of auscultation. Among these has been the development of echocardiography to the extent that this almost constitutes a specialty in its own right. Echocardiography when combined with phonocardiography has provided a hitherto unparalleled opportunity for non-invasive study of the origin and behaviour of heart sounds and murmurs, thereby confirming many of the theories and hypotheses current at the time of writing the last edition and refuting others.

The late Dr Paul Wood in his inspired teaching of auscultation placed great emphasis on the importance of the correlation of physiological and anatomical information with the auscultatory findings. The increase in recent years in non-invasive methods of obtaining this information makes this all the more important. It is therefore particularly appropriate that this edition marks the introduction as co-author of Ronald Gold who was senior registrar to Paul Wood at the Brompton Hospital at the time of his tragically early death. Dr Gold and I have had many stimulating discussions on auscultation over the years and I am delighted that with his enthusiasm and exceptional expertise in the subject he has agreed to join me and to take over as the principal author for the next edition. The task of largely rewriting the text together with the introduction of new material has been mainly his responsibility. To accompany the extensive revision the illustrations have been redrawn and a number of new ones added. We are indebted to David Houghton and Ray Joyce for the meticulous art work this has involved.

Where relevant the echocardiogram has been introduced and increased emphasis has been placed on the correlation between heart sounds and murmurs and the accompanying haemodynamic events. A convention has been adopted under which left heart events are shown in red and those from the right heart in black.

The opportunity has been taken to extend the scope of this book, originally intended for undergraduates alone, to provide for the needs of those who wish for a somewhat more advanced knowledge of the subject, yet still catering for the student who needs to obtain a basic knowledge of the subject. Auscultation is of necessity dealt with all too cursorily in many of the general text books of cardiology. Because of this and the plethora of books now available on echocardiography, the student may be forgiven if he has gained the mistaken idea that a good knowledge of auscultation is no longer necessary. There is a need to bridge the deepening gulf between modern technology on one hand and the British tradition of bedside medicine on the other. The ability to correlate the information obtained from both of these sources leads to a better understanding of and a greater reliance on physical signs. It is hoped that the present edition will fulfil these aims and demonstrate that auscultation continues to be a useful science rather than a lost art.

1984 R.W.D.T.

Contents

1

Observation and palpation

The introduction of laboratory investigations of many kinds has tended to be associated with less thorough bedside examination at which former generations were more practised. On the other hand the accuracy of certain observations has been increased by the introduction of special techniques which have also clarified the meaning of physical signs.

Some physicians are better observers than others and some take more care. This is often a reflection of varying standards of training received by students. This in turn depends on the emphasis the individual teacher places on the present-day importance of a thorough grounding in bedside examination techniques. 'One sees what one knows,' that is to say, the physician is more likely to detect disorders and their associated physical signs, with which he is familiar.

OBSERVATION

Many general observations are relevant to heart disease and a remarkable amount of useful information may be gained by the use of the eyes alone. In the following paragraphs reference is mainly confined to observations which may assist the accurate and full interpretation of auscultatory findings of practical importance. Significant features include age, sex, anxiety, dyspnoea, pain, cough, hoarseness, flushing, pallor, cyanosis, jaundice, obesity, loss of weight, oedema and shock.

Particular attention should be paid to eyes, neck, hands and skin, to deformities such as sternal depression, kyphoscoliosis and spondylosis, and to general conditions such as pregnancy, hyperthyroidism, hypothroidism, rheumatoid arthritis, scleroderma, gout, Cushing's syndrome, Marfan's syndrome and neuromuscular disorders. Alcoholism may be suspected from the face and demeanour.

Certain congenital disorders, such as Down's syndrome (mongolism), are frequently associated with heart disease.

Age and sex may be significant in that certain diseases more frequently occur in particular age groups and in one or other sex. The facial appearance may suggest the diagnosis of an important associated condition almost at a glance, for example the 'pug face' of hypercalcaemia of infancy and supravalvar aortic stenosis.

If the patient can be observed during an attack of pain it is often possible to determine the cause, and likewise that of dyspnoea which may take several forms including orthopnea, hyperpnoea, pulmonary oedema, Cheyne-Stokes respiration and hysterical hyperventilation.

Pregnancy, owing to the increase in cardiac output and circulating blood volume, may be responsible for symptoms and signs which simulate heart disease or may aggravate existing heart disease.

Hyperkinetic circulatory states due to anxiety, fever, pregnancy, anaemia, thyrotoxicosis, chronic hypoxia, advanced liver disease or any form of arteriovenous aneurysm may produce circulatory disturbances including tachycardia, a raised jugular venous pressure, increased praecordial impulses and loudness of heart murmurs and a variety of symptoms, as well as aggravating the symptoms and physical signs of any pre-existing cardiovascular disease.

Anaemia from whatever cause will aggravate symptoms and its correction may relieve cardiac failure or pain. Sometimes however it may be *due* to heart disease as in infective endo-carditis or acute rheumatic fever.

Cough may be due to pulmonary oedema or related to pulmonary heart disease.

Cyanosis, if of central origin, limits the diagnostic field but if of peripheral origin usually reflects only a low cardiac output.

Jaundice may be due to hepatic congestion from cardiac failure, pulmonary infarction or, of course, a non-cardiac cause.

Sweating may be due to anxiety (cold hands), hyperthy-roidism (warm hands) or infection.

Shock may be of cardiac or non-cardiac origin and the cause must be determined.

Fever from any cause, and particularly when due to respir-atory infection, may precipitate cardiac failure. Unexplained fever may be due to thrombophlebitis or pulmonary infarction. If the cause of fever is not obvious in a patient who also has a murmur, infective endocarditis must be excluded as a first priority.

The classical mitral facies consists of high coloured cheeks with a blue tinge due to stagnation of blood in dilated subcu-taneous venules and excessive extraction of oxygen. It is now less often seen and is characteristic of severe mitral disease especially if there is tricuspid regurgitation. It results from a low cardiac output and sluggish peripheral circulation usually with systemic venous hypertension. A similar appearance is only rarely seen in patients with a low output from other causes, presumably because of the relatively short duration of their condition.

Examination of the eyes may show a premature arcus senilis or xanthelasma suggesting hypercholesterolaemia, petechial haemorrhages suggesting infective endocarditis, Argyll-Robertson pupils from syphilitic infection, or Horner's syndrome.

The tongue may be pale from anaemia or show evidence of glossitis, but of greater diagnostic value is the blue discolouration of central cyanosis which is usually best recognised in this situation. Macroglossia may be due to amyloidosis which is one of the less common causes of cardiomyopathy.

The heart may be involved in a variety of systemic diseases including rheumatoid arthritis, systemic sclerosis (scleroderma), disseminated lupus erythematosus, ankylosing spondylitis, neuromuscular disorders and various less common conditions.

Skeletal deformities, as discussed below, may be responsible for apparent cardiac enlargement or be a factor in the aetiology of pulmonary disease.

Inspection and palpation of the neck, anterior chest wall and abdomen and examination of the hands will be discussed in detail.

PALPATION

Knowledge of the fact that there are at least fifty useful physical signs which may be detected by palpation in relation to the cardiovascular system should encourage the student to be methodical. With the advent of more elaborate techniques, clinical methods, including palpation, tend to be neglected and in consequence not only is important information often missed but unnecessary investigations may be carried out.

Bedside cardiology has the enormous advantages of availability, simplicity, safety and absence of pain or even discomfort. Confidence rather than anxiety is engendered by the personal touch.

In recent years instrumental methods, such as impulse cardiography, have established the reliability of the information which can be obtained by simpler techniques.

Attention should be directed towards the chest wall, the neck, the abdomen and the peripheral pulses.

INSPECTION AND PALPATION OF THE NECK

The following points may be of particular importance under varying circumstances:

Differentiation between jugular and carotid pulsations
Jugular venous pressure and pulse
Carotid pulsations
Carotid timing of cardiac events
Effects of carotid compression on heart rate
Carotid massage to terminate paroxysmal tachycardia
Carotid sinus hypersensitivity in cases of syncope
Carotid thrill
Kinking of carotid artery
Goitre

Inspection and palpation of the neck with particular reference to the jugular venous pressure and pulse and to carotid pulsation, should precede auscultation. The presence of a goitre may be of cardiological importance.

Differentiation between carotid and venous pulsation

An inexperienced observer may find difficulty in distinguishing carotid from jugular pulsations, but with practice this is easily accomplished.

In the first place, an arterial pulsation is usually a single, brisk, localised and palpable thrust, whereas a venous pulsation is more gentle and diffuse and in sinus rhythm usually has a double peak.

Palpation of the vessel is not always reliable because, occasionally, a vigorous presystolic venous wave may be easily felt.

Next, an arterial pulse is unaffected by respiration, posture or pressure over the abdomen whereas a venous pulse normally decreases with inspiration or sitting up and, conversely, is exaggerated with expiration, lying down and abdominal pressure.

Finally, if the *external* jugular vein is compressed in the supraclavicular fossa the vein will fill from above, and can be emptied by compression higher in the neck with release of the compression lower down. Light pressure will obliterate or markedly reduce venous, but not arterial pulsation.

JUGULAR VENOUS PRESSURE AND PULSE

Close inspection and measurement of the jugular venous pressure and pulse may give very important information and sometimes the first lead to a correct diagnosis.

Jugular venous pressure

The examination should be made under optimal conditions with suitable. preferably oblique lighting. The patient should be comfortable and relaxed reclining first at an angle of about 45° (Fig. 1b), but subsequent adjustment of this angle may be

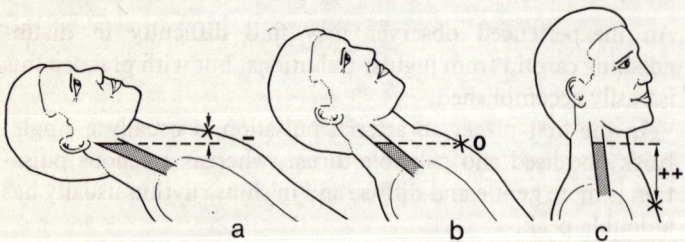

Fig. 1 Examination and measurement of the jugular venous pulse. For observation of the jugular venous pulse, variation in posture from almost supine (a) to almost upright (c) is necessary depending on the height of the jugular venous pressure. In patients with a normal or only mildly raised jugular venous pressure this is best observed at an angle of about 45° (b). The pressure is measured vertically using the sternal angle (x) as the zero reference.

necessary to render the peaks of the venous pulsation clearly visible. If the pressure is markedly elevated an almost upright posture may be needed (Fig. 1c) whereas if the jugular pulse is not obvious above the clavicles the patient may have to lie flatter (Fig. 1a). Patients often try to help by hyperextending the neck. While a moderate degree of elevation of the chin may be helpful, too much tenses the tissues of the neck and may make examination more difficult.

The pressure is measured as the *vertical* distance from the sternal angle to the peak of pulsation at the end of expiration during quiet steady breathing (Fig. 2), *never* with held respiration as this may be accompanied by closure of the glottis and a sharp rise in intrathoracic pressure, producing falsely high readings. It is wise to record also the angle of inclination of the patient as some variation in jugular venous pressure can occur with changes in posture. The normal jugular venous pressure should be not more than 2 cm above the sternal angle with the patient at 45°.

Both sides of the neck should be examined because there

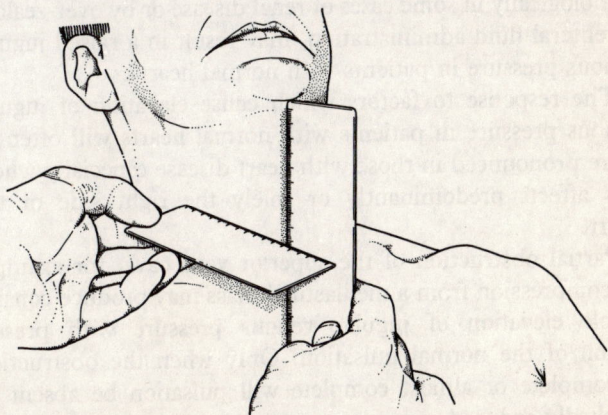

Fig. 2 Measurement of the jugular venous pressure.

may be differences. It is the deeply situated internal vein, which cannot be directly observed, that provides most information and acts as a convenient manometer of central (right atrial) venous pressure.

The characteristic 'welling' pulsation can readily be detected by the experienced observer but is frequently missed if attention is confined to the superficial external jugular veins. These veins are often obstructed as they pass through the fascial planes and are therefore an unreliable guide to venous pressure and pulsation.

The venous pressure may be significantly raised by anxiety, a fact which explains why this is sometimes evident at first examination in the consulting room or outpatient clinic, but not thereafter. The explanation lies in a redistribution of blood from vasoconstriction of the capacitance vessels. Likewise a hyperkinetic circulatory state from any cause may produce elevation of jugular venous pressure in a patient with a normal heart.

An increased blood volume, occurring physiologically in women during the premenstrual phase and in pregnancy, or pathologically in some cases of renal disease or by over-zealous parenteral fluid administration, may result in a raised jugular venous pressure in patients with normal hearts.

The response to factors which cause elevation of jugular venous pressure in patients with normal hearts will often be more pronounced in those with heart disease especially where this affects predominantly or solely the right side of the heart.

Partial obstruction of the superior vena cava, for example by compression from a mediastinal mass may produce considerable elevation of jugular venous pressure with preservation of the normal pulsation. Only when the obstruction is complete or almost complete will pulsation be absent or markedly reduced.

Where the raised jugular venous pressure reflects an

increased right atrial pressure due to heart disease, this will be due to one or more of the following mechanisms:

1. Impaired emptying of the right atrium from tricuspid valve stenosis.
2. Increased resistance to filling of the right ventricle from cardiac failure.
3. Tricuspid regurgitation.
4. Reduced distensibility of right heart from cardiac tamponade or pericardial constriction.

Effect of respiration

The effect of deep, slow respiration on the jugular venous pressure should be observed. In health and in most patients with heart disease the venous pressure falls on inspiration due to the increased negativity of the intrathoracic pressure which facilitates venous return to the right heart.

During coughing or the Valsalva manoeuvre, the sharp increase in intrathoracic pressure impedes the return of venous blood to the right heart resulting in transient quite marked elevation of jugular venous pressure.

In patients with cardiac tamponade or constrictive pericarditis and in some patients with right heart failure there may be a paradoxical rise in jugular venous pressure with inspiration (Kussmaul's sign). This is due to further impairment of right heart filling when the pericardial tension is increased by the descent of the diaphragm with inspiration.

Jugular venous pulsation

In addition to the measurement of the jugular venous pressure, analysis of the individual waves of the jugular venous pulse which with practice is possible in most patients at the bedside can provide valuable diagnostic information.

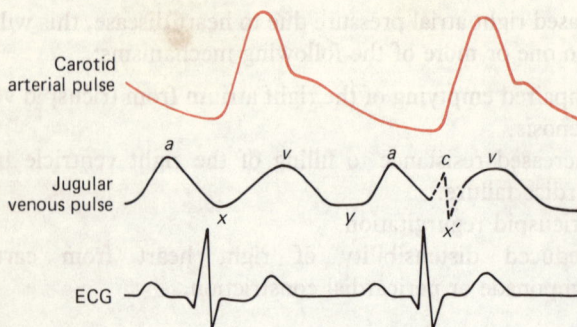

Fig. 3 The normal jugular venous and carotid arterial pulses.

The jugular venous pulse nomally consists of four waves, *a*, *x*, *v* and *y* (Fig. 3).

The *a* wave is a positive wave due to right atrial systole. It disappears in atrial fibrillation.

The *x* descent (systolic collapse) is the negative wave which follows immediately the *a* wave and is due mainly to atrial relaxation and also disappears in atrial fibrillation.

The *v* wave is the second positive wave which represents the rise in right atrial pressure as this fills during ventricular systole. It reaches its peak at the end of systole.

The *y* descent (diastolic collapse) is the negative wave which follows *v* and is due to the fall in right atrial pressure on opening of the tricuspid valve.

A third positive wave, the *c* wave is described but is rarely visible on clinical examination. It interrupts the *x* descent and is probably due to closure of the tricuspid valve rather than to a transmitted carotid pulsation.

The abnormal wave due to tricuspid regurgitation is not an exaggeration of the normal *v* wave but occurs earlier in systole, and directly after or replacing the *x* descent. It should therefore not be described as a *v* wave, as is commonly done, but as an *s* (systolic) wave (Fig. 4). Tricuspid regurgitation is present in many patients with severe cardiac failure.

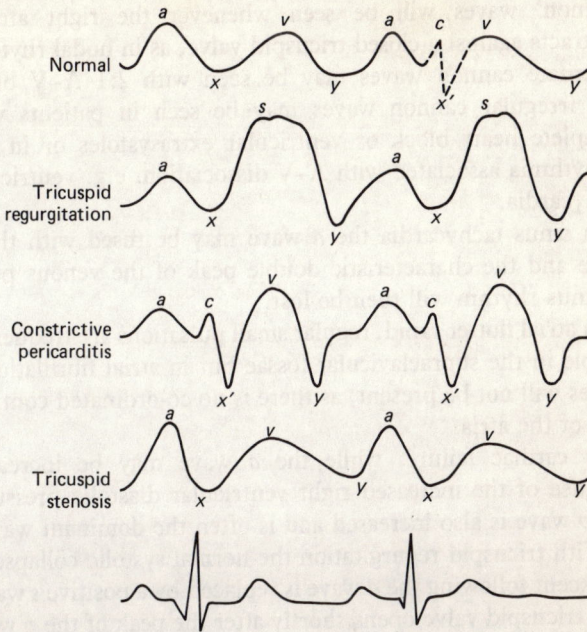

Fig. 4 The jugular venous pulse wave in health and disease.

In health presystolic *a* is usually the largest positive wave (Fig. 4). An exaggerated or single 'giant' *a* wave may be present if emptying of the right atrium during contraction is impeded either by tricuspid stenosis, a closed tricuspid valve, the so-called 'cannon' wave, or decreased right ventricular compliance due to hypertrophy from whatever cause. Under these conditions the *a* wave has a characteristic sharp-peaked 'flicking' quality and may be so vigorous as to be mistaken for an arterial pulsation.

In the presence of sinus rhythm, the detection of a prominent presystolic wave may provide the first clue to the presence of tricuspid stenosis and, if this is missed, other signs may be unrecognised or misinterpreted. Regular exaggerated or 'cannon' waves will be seen whenever the right atrium contracts against a closed tricuspid valve, as in nodal rhythm. Alternate cannon waves may be seen with 2:1 A–V block and irregular cannon waves may be seen in patients with complete heart block or ventricular extrasystoles or in any arrhythmia associated with A–V dissociation, e.g. ventricular tachycardia.

In sinus tachycardia the *a* wave may be fused with the *v* wave and the characteristic double peak of the venous pulse in sinus rhythm will then be lost.

In atrial flutter rapid, regular small pulsations are frequently visible in the supraclavicular fossae but in atrial fibrillation *a* waves will not be present, as there is no co-ordinated contraction of the atria.

In cardiac failure, while the *a* wave may be increased because of the increased right ventricular diastolic pressure, the *v* wave is also increased and is often the dominant wave.

With tricuspid regurgitation the normal systolic collapse or *x* descent following the *a* wave is replaced by a positive *s* wave. The tricuspid valve opens shortly after the peak of the *v* wave immediately following the second heart sound, and the *y* descent represents the phase of rapid, right ventricular filling from the atrium (Fig. 4).

Numerous factors influence the *y* descent, including the height of the venous pressure, the pressure-volume characteristics of the right atrium and ventricle, and the presence of tricuspid stenosis. Prominent diastolic collapse is a feature of tricuspid regurgitation and may be the most striking abnormality to be observed in the jugular venous pulse. Conversely in severe tricuspid stenosis the slow emptying of the right atrium produces a slower than normal *y* descent (Fig. 4).

In cardiac tamponade and early constrictive pericarditis the dominant negative wave may be systolic in timing (Fig. 4). Unlike the normal *x* descent it is still seen in patients with atrial fibrillation and is known as the *x'* descent. In patients with sinus rhythm it is sometimes distinguishable from the normal x descent from which it is separated by a small c wave. In advanced constrictive pericarditis the dominant negative wave is the y descent as in cardiac failure.

Carotid pulse

The carotid, rather than the radial pulse, is the best guide to timing of auscultatory events in the cardiac cycle. Exaggerated carotid pulsation is most frequently due to aortic regurgitation with a large left ventricular stroke volume. This was first reported by Corrigan who, incidentally, made no reference to the corresponding collapsing radial pulse as commonly thought.

Excessive pulsation may also result from coarctation of the aorta, in which case the femoral pulse will be weak and delayed after the radial.

In hypertension from other causes the pulsation is usually normal. Absent or unequal pulsations on the two sides usually result from atherosclerosis and this sign may be of value in the analysis of cerebral symptoms. Rarely it results from embolism or from obstruction due to a dissecting aneurysm of the aorta. In this context it may be noted that a carotid systolic thrill may have a similar significance.

In severe aortic stenosis the pulse is usually of small volume and slow-rising (anacrotic).

A double (bisferiens) pulse is often present with a combination of aortic stenosis and regurgitation.

Carotid compression may be used to slow the heart rate and thus facilitate timing in auscultation, to separate the two components of gallop rhythm, to terminate an attack of supraventricular tachycardia or temporarily change the degree of block in atrial flutter, or to confirm or exclude that hypersensitivity of the carotid sinus may be the cause of syncopal attacks or dizziness.

Carotid sinus pressure and massage

If light pressure over the carotid sinus does not influence the heart beat, firm massage up and down should be begun and maintained whilst counting mentally up to a maximum of about 10 seconds. A change of rhythm or cardiac arrest can be seen on the e.c.g., detected at the radial pulse or noted on auscultation.

There may be no effect, the paroxysm may be terminated, or the heart rate may be temporarily slowed. Cardiac arrest may occur and continue whilst pressure is maintained. If pressure is kept up for too long, syncope and convulsions may follow, but this of course should be avoided.

Correctly applied vagal stimulation by carotid sinus massage is often effective and the administration of drugs or electrical countershock rendered unnecessary. However, only paroxysmal atrial or AV junctional (nodal) tachycardia is likely to be arrested. There will be no effect on ventricular tachycardia. In sinus tachycardia the rate may be temporarily slowed and in atrial flutter the degree of block is often transiently increased.

Kinked carotid

A localised vigorous pulsation above the right clavicle may be due to kinking of the carotid artery from atherosclerosis, usually in association with a high aortic arch from unfolding. This condition may simulate an innominate aneurysm, which is relatively rare, but can usually be distinguished by palpation.

ARTERIAL PULSE

No examination of the cardiovascular system is complete without the palpation of all peripheral arterial pulses, especially where peripheral vascular disease or arterial dissection is suspected. In the normal subject it is nearly always possible to detect on each side of the body the carotid, subclavian, axillary, brachial, radial, femoral, popliteal, dorsalis pedis and posterior tibial pulses. Each pulse should be compared with the corresponding pulse on the opposite side of the body and any inequality in volume or timing should be noted.

Unequal pulsations

Unequal arterial pulsations are most often due to narrowing or obstruction from atherosclerosis but may also result from systemic embolism, congenital malformation, or surgical procedures such as arterial catheterisation or Blalock (subclavian-pulmonary artery) anastomosis.

A particular example of unequal pulses is the subclavian 'steal' sydrome in which narrowing or occlusion is responsible for vertebral arterial insufficiency with cerebral symptoms, sometimes aggravated by using the arm on that side. However, this interesting condition properly belongs to the domain of peripheral vascular disease.

Every cardiological examination should include simultaneous palpation of radial and femoral arteries. Failure to do so will sooner or later result in the otherwise easily clinically diagnosed condition of coarctation of the aorta being missed. Normally the radial and femoral arteries are synchronous in timing and approximately equal in volume. Noticeable delay and reduction in volume of femoral artery pulsation are characteristic findings of coarctation. Before comparing radial and femoral pulsations it is important to ascertain that both radial artery pulses are equal and synchronous as occasionally the coarctation is proximal to the origin of the left subclavian artery. In such a case left radial and both femoral artery pulses will be diminished and delayed equally, so that the diagnosis may be missed.

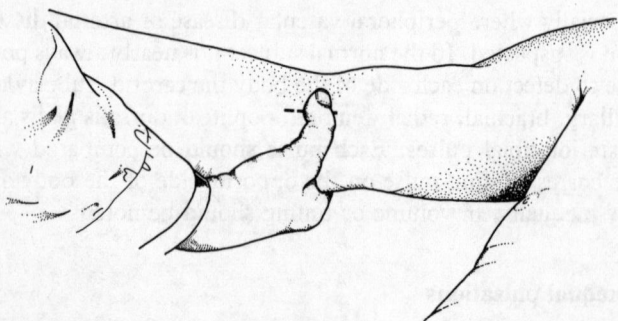

Fig. 5 Palpation of the brachial arterial pulse.

Where narrowing or obstruction of an artery is suspected, auscultation over the artery (Fig. 5) should be carried out to detect the presence of a continuous murmur (see p. 142).

FEATURES OF THE ARTERIAL PULSE

In the past, great emphasis was placed on the ritual of palpation of the radial pulse. Today this is still expected by most patients and it does establish initial contact with the patient and often instils confidence. However, the radial artery is too small a vessel and too peripherally placed to afford much reliable information.

The pulse wave travels from the heart via a branching system of tubes with elastic walls. This gives rise to a complex interaction of reflected waves with the main pulse wave producing a higher systolic and lower diastolic pressure in the smaller peripheral arteries than in the proximal aorta. At the same time the wave form becomes smoothed out, obliterating changes in its rate of rise and fall. The carotid arteries afford the most proximal position from which to palpate the arterial wave form but proper examination of this requires application of a variable but considerable amount of pressure over the vessel. If one uses the carotid artery, this can be difficult for the examiner and uncomfortable for the patient. The most convenient artery to examine, which is still large enough and central enough to provide reliable information, is the brachial artery.

Palpation of the brachial artery

A right-handed physician will normally carry out clinical examination from the patient's right side. In this case the right brachial artery should be palpated by the right hand of the examiner. A left-handed examiner may prefer to approach the patient from the left side and palpate the left brachial artery with his left hand. The patient's elbow is cradled in the palm of the examiner's hand. In this position the examiner's thumb comes to lie automatically over the brachial artery (Fig. 5). Pressure is then applied progressively by the thumb over the artery so as to explore the whole of the arterial wave from peak to trough. Too light a pressure will detect only the peak of the arterial pulse and will not allow appreciation of the rate of rise and fall of the pulse wave and any change in rate. The use of the thumb with its greater tactile area than any of the fingers enables the examiner to apply and vary the pressure on the artery more evenly and more easily sense the underlying pressure wave.

Pulse rate

When the rhythm is regular and the rate not excessively fast the pulse rate provides an accurate measure of heart rate. However when the rhythm is irregular, heart beats preceded by a short diastolic filling period may produce insufficient stroke output for the resultant pulse wave to be palpable. The same difficulty occurs when the cardiac output is low and at very high heart rates even in regular rhythm. In these cases simultaneous observation of the heart rate by auscultation and the peripheral pulse rate produces a difference known as the *pulse deficit*. This will be greatest with fast irregular rhythms such as uncontrolled atrial fibrillation and will gradually disappear as the rhythm is brought under control. However its estimation is of very dubious value. Of much more practical value is the accurate recording of heart rate by the only reliable means of measuring it under these conditions, i.e. by auscultation of the heart.

In regular rhythm it is sufficient to count the pulse for 15 seconds and multiply the result by four to give the heart rate. Where the rhythm is irregular or there is bradycardia the period of observation should be extended to 30 seconds or 1 minute.

Rates between 50 and 130 at rest, are usually physiological but these limits may be exceeded.

A rate greater than 140/minute, when not due to exertion, emotion or fever, is usually due to an ectopic pacemaker, that is to say, one outside the SA node, and attention should be paid to the jugular venous pulse, the heart sounds and the effect of carotid sinus massage as described above. A rate below 50/minute is due to heart block but may result from sinus bradycardia.

The most frequent causes of an irregular pulse are sinus arrhythmia, extrasystoles and atrial fibrillation. Other causes include atrial flutter or atrial tachycardia with varying block and dropped beats from impaired conduction.

Volume and character of the arterial pulse

These two qualities of the arterial pulse wave are inseparable and alterations in the volume of the pulse can materially affect the character of the pulse wave and the recognition of abnormalities of its character. Both are affected by a number of factors, in particular the calibre of the vessel palpated, the cardiac output, the force of left ventricular contraction, the presence of obstruction to the outflow tract of the left ventricle and of aortic or mitral regurgitation and the peripheral arterial resistance. The brachial pulse, examined carefully as outlined above, provides the most convenient and reliable pulse for clinical assessment of these features. The radial pulse is too peripheral and too small and is unreliable.

In general a pulse of small volume reflects a low LV stroke volume and a bounding pulse with a normal upstroke indicates an increased LV stroke volume and is seen characteristically in any of the hyperkinetic circulatory states, including that due to nervousness of the patient. Beat by beat variation of the pulse volume will occur with irregular rhythms, due to the effect of the varying duration of the preceding diastolic filling period of the left ventricle on the force of left ventricular contraction.

In *pulsus alternans* regular larger and smaller beats alternate. The mechanism of this is not well understood but it is usually associated with impaired left ventricular function. It is often best appreciated by sphygmomanometry, when a difference of up to 20 mmHg may be found in the systolic pressure between alternate beats.

An even larger alternation of pulse volume is seen in *pulsus bigeminus* due to ventricular ectopic beats occurring alternately with normal beats (Fig. 6). The earlier the ectopic beat occurs the shorter will be the preceding diastolic filling period for that beat which will consequently be reduced in volume, sometimes to an extent which makes it barely palpable at the brachial pulse and impalpable at the radial pulse. Conversely because of the increased diastolic filling period due to the compensatory pause following the ventricular ectopic beat, the normal beats are of increased volume. Palpation of the radial pulse in such cases may give rise to a wrong diagnosis of bradycardia and auscultation is necessary to reveal the true situation.

Pulsus paradoxus is a term in common use but a misnomer in that it reflects exaggeration of the normal respiratory vari-

ARTERIAL PULSE

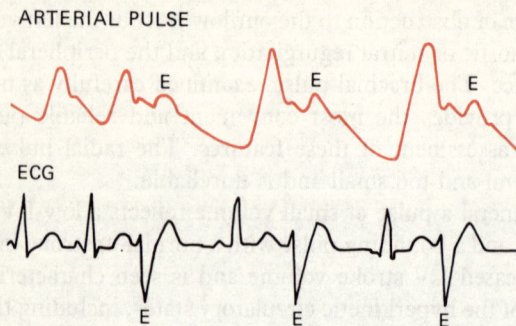

Fig. 6 Pulsus bigeminus. The arterial pulse wave resulting from the ventricular ectopic beat (E) is small or even impalpable.

ation in systolic pressure. In healthy persons this is rarely perceptible by palpation of the arterial pulse, although systolic pressure may be decreased by 5 or even 10 mmHg with inspiration.

If suspected, confirmation should be sought by measuring the blood pressure. If the cuff is inflated until sounds can no longer be heard over the brachial artery and the pressure then allowed gradually to fall, it will first be noted that sounds are audible only in expiration. With a further fall in pressure, sounds will be heard throughout the respiratory cycle and, by convention, if the difference between the two readings exceeds 10 mmHg pulsus paradoxus is said to be present.

Pulsus paradoxus may result from rapid accumulation of a pericardial effusion, from constrictive pericarditis or restrictive cardiomyopathy. It may, however, also result from any condition causing wide fluctuations in intrathoracic pressure, such as obstructive airway disease or the stiff lungs of pulmonary venous congestion.

The phenomenon of pulsus paradoxus is an exaggeration of the normal response to respiration. In normal subjects return of blood from the lungs to the left heart is reduced on inspiration probably because the negative intrathoracic pressure and expansion of the lungs increases the capacity of the pulmonary vascular bed. This is normally partly offset by an increase in right ventricular output on inspiration due to the increased venous return to the right heart produced by the negative intrathoracic pressure. In pericardial tamponade and constriction the limitation of filling of the right ventricle with inspiration means that this increase in right ventricular output does not occur and the filling of left ventricle on inspiration is consequently less than in the normal subject, thus reducing the pulse volume on inspiration.

The quality of the brachial pulse is something which can only be learned by practice and experience. It is important to learn to recognise what the normal pulse wave feels like. Attention should be directed in turn to its upstroke, peak and downstroke. The upstroke of the normal pulse wave is smooth and fairly rapid with a uniform rate of rise (slope) throughout (Fig. 7a). Its peak is momentarily sustained and is followed by the downstroke, the initial part of which has approximately the same slope as the upstroke. In the normal subject it is not usually possible to appreciate the dicrotic notch or the much slower falling part of the downstroke beyond it. However when considerable vasodilatation is present, resulting in the circulating blood volume becoming smaller relative to the increased volume of the vascular bed available for filling, the initial fairly rapid part of the downstroke continues further down from the peak and is interrupted by a palpable dicrotic notch which is sometimes followed by a small positive pressure wave (the dicrotic wave) as in Figure 7b. This so-called *dicrotic pulse* is found chiefly in patients in whom fever is accompanied by vasodilatation and occasionally in conditions associated with a reduced circulatory blood volume unaccompanied by a fall in cardiac output or reflex peripheral vasoconstriction. It is not an indication of any cardiac abnormality.

The *bounding pulse* which is seen characteristically in any of

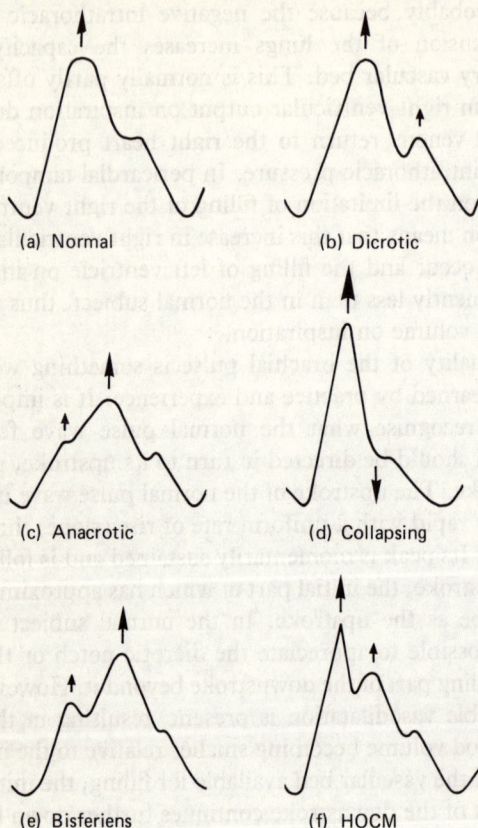

(a) Normal

(b) Dicrotic

(c) Anacrotic

(d) Collapsing

(e) Bisferiens

(f) HOCM

Fig. 7 Normal and abnormal arterial pulse waves. The arrows indicate the direction and magnitude of the palpable impulses. HOCM = Hypertrophic obstructive cardiomyopathy.

the hyperkinetic circulatory states is simply a variation of the normal pulse brought about by a high pulse pressure associated with increased blood flow. Its wave form is quite normal.

The presence of a slow upstroke of the brachial pulse wave associated with some reduction in pulse amplitude can with practice usually be identified except where the pulse is of small volume due to a low cardiac output. With careful palpation a change in slope of the upstroke can often be appreciated. This *anacrotic shoulder* divides the upstroke approximately into two halves, the upper being slower rising than the lower initial half (Fig. 7c). This *anacrotic pulse* is characteristic of aortic stenosis of at least moderate severity. Lesser degrees of aortic stenosis may not produce a recognisable degree of slowing of the upstroke. Severe aortic stenosis may however be present especially in children without an anacrotic pulse. In aortic stenosis complicated by heart failure the pulse may be too small for its anacrotic nature to be recognised.

A steeply rising pulse with a sharp peak and an equally rapid downstroke is known as a *collapsing pulse* or *water-hammer pulse* (Fig. 7d). The slope of its upstroke is steep and uniform from onset to peak. The pulse pressure (the difference between systolic and diastolic blood pressure) is increased, principally due to a low diastolic pressure although the systolic blood pressure may also be increased if the left ventricle is ejecting a larger volume of blood than normal. The collapsing pulse is typical of severe aortic regurgitation but is also found in patent ductus, arteriovenous fistula or in any condition in which peripheral resistance is lowered by a leak from the arterial side of the circulation. A collapsing pulse is also found in severe mitral regurgitation but in this condition the amplitude of the pulse is usually lower because of the reduced forward flow during left ventricular systole. A collapsing pulse is occasionally found in conditions associated with generalised rigidity and loss of elasticity of the large arteries as in syphilitic aortitis.

In combined aortic stenosis and regurgitation the pulse wave presents some of the features of each condition. The initial upstroke is slower than normal though steeper than in aortic stenosis. The anacrotic shoulder is more pronounced and occurs higher on the upstroke of the pulse. It is often so pronounced as to feel almost equal in amplitude to the peak of the pulse (Fig. 7e). This 'twice-beating' pulse is known as *pulsus bisferiens*. If inadequate pressure is used in palpating the artery only the second true peak will be appreciated and the bisferiens nature of the pulse will be missed.

In *hypertrophic obstructive cardiomyopathy* (HOCM) of the left ventricle the pulse is 'jerky' in character due to a very abrupt upstroke which consists of the percussion wave. The tidal wave is much delayed and occurs on the downstroke of the pulse. In severe hypertrophic obstructive cardiomyopathy this delayed tidal peak may be palpable and may be mistaken for a dicrotic wave but it occurs earlier and is more sustained than the latter (Fig. 7f).

In a patient with coarctation of the aorta, unequal pulses suggest that the obstruction is proximal to the left subclavian artery.

EXAMINATION OF THE HANDS

Whilst palpating the arterial pulse for rate, rhythm and quality, the opportunity should be taken to examine the hands for features which may be relevant to heart disease.

Long, slender fingers (arachnodactyly) may be normal and sometimes occurs in families but also as part of the Marfan syndrome which includes cardiovascular manifestations such as dilatation of the aorta, aortic regurgitation, rupture of the aorta and various congenital cardiac anomalies.

Cold moist hands suggest anxiety, warm moist hands thyrotoxicosis and dry hands with a rough skin the possibility of hypothyroidism.

Unusually warm hands may be present with any high output state and cold hands with a low output.

Cyanosis is likely to be central in origin if the hands are warm, in which case it will also be obvious in the tongue. If the hands are cold and the tongue is pink cyanosis will be of peripheral origin, and the arterial oxygen saturation normal.

Central cyanosis in a child and the association of central cyanosis with clubbing of the fingers is usually due to congenital heart disease.

Clubbing of the fingers in a patient with heart disease may be due to infective endocarditis, a right to left shunt or some associated but unrelated condition. Clubbing may also be a sign of postoperative infection, particularly after open heart surgery.

Anaemia may be obvious in the nails and if koilonychia is present iron deficiency is likely to be the cause. Whatever the cause, anaemia is harmful to those with heart disease and should be corrected. This may result, for example, in the relief of cardiac failure or of cardiac pain. Anaemia is usually present in infective endocarditis and acute rheumatic fever.

Splinter haemorrhages under the nails may be due to infective endocarditis but may be seen in otherwise healthy patients with valvar disease and are not uncommon in normal individuals, particularly manual workers.

Osler's nodes are painful, tender, reddish-brown areas in the pads of the fingers. They are uncommon but characteristic of infective endocarditis.

Rheumatic nodules are more commonly present over the occiput or elbows but may occur on the tendon sheaths in front of the wrists. In their presence active myocarditis can be presumed.

Rheumatoid nodules may suggest the cause of apparently idiopathic pericarditis. Systolic murmurs may also be present from involvement of the endocardium. Rheumatoid nodules may be present on the hands but more often near the elbows.

Gout is another form of arthritis which is occasionally associated with pericarditis. The feet should also be examined, and the hands for tophi.

There is probably a higher incidence of coronary disease in persons with hyperuricaemia.

Scleroderma (systemic sclerosis) may involve the fingers and be associated with myocardial fibrosis, pericarditis or, in advanced cases, cardiac failure.

Xanthomata may be observed as orange-yellow tinged streaks in the palms, as nodules over tendon sheaths or as raised eruptions in the skin. They suggest hyperlipidaemia which is often present with coronary atherosclerosis.

'*Liver palms*' may be due to cirrhosis of the liver in association with heart disease. However, palmar erythema is a non-specific sign.

Capillary pulsation, which is best seen in the nail beds after light pressure, is an unimportant sign of aortic regurgitation because, when present, there will always be more obvious manifestations and at an earlier stage. It may occur with peripheral vasodilatation with warm hands from any cause, such as a hot bath.

PALPATION OF THE ANTERIOR CHEST WALL

Apex beat

Position
  Displacement of heart
  Cardiac enlargement
Character
  Left ventricular hypertrophy — hyperdynamic impulse
  Left ventricular dilatation — hyperkinetic impulse
  Double impulse
  Tapping impulse
  Triple rhythm
  Impalpable impulse
Thrills
  Mitral regurgitation
  Mitral stenosis

Anterior ventricular wall

Right ventricular hypertrophy
Right ventricular dilatation
Myocardial dysfunction
Ventricular aneurysm
Left atrial expansion
Thrills
   Ventricular septal defect

Basal region

Pulmonary hypertension
   Pulmonary arterial lift
   Pulmonary valve closure
Thrills
   Aortic stenosis
   Pulmonary stenosis
   Patent ductus

Miscellaneous

Dilatation of aorta
Collateral vessels

Palpation should be carried out according to an accustomed and systematic regime, as with auscultation.

The patient should be supine and comfortably reclining on a bed or couch at an angle of about 30°. The observer should sit on the patient's right and apply the palmar surface of the right hand systematically to the region of the apical impulse, the sternum, the parasternal areas, the base of the heart and the epigastrium. A localised pulsation should be palpated with the finger tips.

After inspection of the chest to determine any abnormal

contour or pulsation, the next step should be to determine the position of the *apex beat*. This is usually defined as the point lowest down and farthest out where the finger is distinctly lifted.

The impulse is normally within the left midclavicular line which usually in males corresponds to the nipple line, and in the fifth intercostal space, but is sometimes in the sixth and occasionally in the fourth space, depending on the position of the diaphragm.

If the position of maximal pulsation is outside the midclavicular line, in the absence of mediastinal displacement from skeletal, pulmonary or pleural causes cardiac enlargement can be diagnosed.

Common causes of displacement to the left are depression of the lower sternum and scoliosis, a fact which emphasises the importance of initial inspection.

Before deciding that the impulse is impalpable, dextrocardia should be excluded by palpation on the opposite side.

The impulse may be impalpable owing to obesity, a thick chest wall from muscular development, a rounded configuration of the chest which increases the distance between the heart and the ribs, emphysema, cardiac failure or constrictive pericarditis. With enlargement of the right ventricle (RV) the whole of the anterior surface of the heart may be formed by the RV which displaces the left ventricular apex away from the chest wall. In such cases the apex beat is ill defined and difficult to localise.

The character of the apex beat is at least as, if not more important than its position. The character of the impulse will be determined by the force of left ventricular contraction, the degree of resistance to expulsion of blood from the ventricle and the volume of blood being ejected.

The normal impulse consists of a brief outward movement at the onset of left ventricular ejection and is probably due to recoil of the heart as a reaction to this.

The amplitude of the apex beat to palpation will vary considerably with the thickness of the chest wall. In normal subjects with a thin chest wall and in patients who have undergone thoracotomy with rib resection, or radical mastectomy, a normal apex beat may appear overactive. Similarly an overactive impulse of normal form may be found in healthy children and in patients with anxiety or hyperkinetic circulatory states such as pregnancy, anaemia or thyrotoxicosis.

The form of the abnormal apex beat differs considerably according to whether the left ventricle (LV) is subject to a volume overload in diastole producing left ventricular dilatation or to a pressure overload in systole producing left ventricular hypertrophy.

In volume overload of the LV as in aortic or mitral regurgitation, ventricular septal defect or patent ductus arteriosus, the dilated ventricle contracts briskly, ejecting blood rapidly against a low resistance. The resulting *hyperkinetic* apex beat is one of increased movement but the contraction is not prolonged.

In pressure overload of the LV as in aortic stenosis or hypertension, the left ventricular hypertrophy (LVH) produces a slow, powerful sustained apical thrust, the *hyperdynamic* apex beat. This term is commonly but wrongly used to describe the hyperkinetic apex beat but in the latter increased movement rather than increased force is the striking feature.

Dilatation and hypertrophy may both be present, as in combined aortic stenosis and regurgitation, and some overlap of the features of the apex beat may occur. In very severe aortic stenosis, rather than the severely hyperdynamic apex beat one would expect, not uncommonly the praecordium is extremely quiet, the apex beat being difficult to feel or even absent.

A central thrust or lift in the sternal region, *best appreciated with the breath held in expiration*, is most often due to right ventricular hypertrophy (RVH) from systolic overload. It may also result from dilatation due to volume overload as from an atrial septal defect. It is often possible to distinguish these two causes but again there may be overlap. In particular, dilatation from increased volume load leads in time to hypertrophy.

A central lift may also be due to systolic expansion of the left atrium from mitral regurgitation. If there is gross dilatation of this chamber there may also be some pulsation to the right of the sternum and a rocking motion of the entire chest wall.

With enlargement of the RV, the heart may be rotated so that the apex is formed by this chamber, but in such cases there will also be a central lift. Likewise, with LV enlargement, this chamber may be responsible, not only for the apical impulse but for a central systolic lift between the apex and the sternum. However, LVH does not cause an isolated central thrust nor RVH an isolated apical one. With biventricular hypertrophy it is usually possible to distinguish two separate systolic thrusts of different qualities.

Palpation is a better guide to ventricular hypertrophy than radiography, which reflects cardiac enlargement but not hypertrophy, and considerable hypertrophy may be present without radiographic enlargement, as in isolated aortic stenosis. Palpation can often also determine better than radiography which ventricle is hypertrophied.

An abnormal outward systolic pulsation to the left of the midsternal region may be felt after acute myocardial infarction or with left ventricular dysfunction during an attack of anginal pain, or from ventricular aneurysm.

A central pulsation is sometimes due to forward displacement of the heart by a pericardial effusion, hiatus hernia, eventration of the diaphragm or mediastinal tumour.

Occasionally the apical impulse is retractile during systole from constrictive pericarditis, tricuspid regurgitation or pleuro-pericardial adhesions.

A 'tapping' apical impulse corresponds to the loud first heart sound in mitral stenosis. It is not related to right ventricular hypertrophy.

Palpable pulmonary valve closure corresponds to a loud pulmonary component of the second sound and is due to pulmonary hypertension.

A palpable third heart sound in early diastole, during the period of rapid ventricular filling, usually reflects ventricular failure.

A pericardial 'knock' early in diastole is due to abrupt limitation of ventricular filling in constrictive pericarditis.

A palpable presystolic impulse corresponding in timing to the fourth heart sound, is due to atrial contraction against an increased ventricular filling resistance.

A double impulse *in systole* is often present in left ventricular hypertrophic obstructive cardiomyopathy but can be difficult to distinguish clinically from the palpable presystolic impulse which also occurs in this condition because of increased left ventricular filling resistance.

Thrills

In the past, too much emphasis was placed on the diagnostic importance of a thrill. A thrill is simply a palpable murmur. Whether a murmur is palpable or not depends not only on its loudness but its character. A harsh, coarse or rumbling murmur is more likely to be palpable than a blowing murmur. The timing of the thrill will of course be that of the underlying murmur.

A basal thrill usually arises from aortic or pulmonary stenosis, an apical systolic thrill from mitral regurgitation and an apical diastolic thrill from mitral stenosis. A left parasternal thrill is most frequently due to a ventricular septal defect.

Sometimes a diffuse systolic thrill with a 'purring' quality arises from rupture of a papillary muscle, and a continuous thrill to the left of the upper sternal border may be due to a patent ductus.

Occasionally a faint sytolic thrill at the left sternal border is due solely to increased pulmonary blood flow, that is from an atrial septal defect, without pulmonary stenosis.

PALPATION OF THE ABDOMEN

Palpation of the abdomen should follow that of the chest, with particular reference to abnormalities relevant to the cardio-vascular system.

Epigastric pulsation may be due to the aorta, right ventricle or liver.

With a hyperkinetic circulation from any cause, including nervousness, or even without this in a thin person, a normal aorta is often palpable. Dilatation of the abdominal aorta is usually due to atherosclerosis with or without aneurysm formation.

A palpable epigastric thrust from right ventricular hyper-trophy usually also causes a lift over the lower sternum.

The liver may be enlarged from cardiac failure or cardiac cirrhosis. Systolic expansion of the liver is a characteristic finding in tricuspid regurgitation. In acute cardiac failure it is likely to be tender, and in cirrhosis it is firm or hard.

The spleen may be enlarged from infective endocarditis or cardiac failure but is occasionally palpable in patients with rheumatic heart disease without these complications. It may also be enlarged in association with hepatic cirrhosis.

Systemic hypertension may be related to renal disease with enlargement of one or both kidneys.

Ascites in the present context suggests cardiac failure usually with cirrhosis of the liver or, less often, constrictive pericar-ditis in which case abdominal enlargement from ascites is frequently disproportionate to the relatively small amount of peripheral oedema.

The femoral pulses may be weak, and delayed after the radial, due to coarctation of the aorta. Either femoral pulse may be weak or impalpable from atherosclerosis, embolism or occasionally a dissecting aneurysm of the aorta.

EXAMINATION OF THE SKELETAL SYSTEM

Various deformities of the spine and chest wall may be significant in relation to heart disease. Important are sternal depression, scoliosis, severe kyphoscoliosis, and a 'straight back' (loss of normal kyphosis).

Scoliosis

Even a mild degree of scoliosis may be responsible for displacement of the apex beat to the left and hence a mistaken diagnosis of cardiac enlargement. This possibility should be suspected on examination from the front, with the individual standing, if the left shoulder and nipple are higher on the left side.

Sternal depression

Funnel- or cup-shaped depression of the sternum is rarely responsible for pulmonary or cardiac disorders but may lead to a mistaken diagnosis of cardiac enlargement from displacement of the apex beat to the left, or of valvar disease from the association of a systolic murmur.

Kyphoscoliosis

Deformities of the spine and thoracic cage may be due to congenital disorders, tuberculosis, rickets, poliomyelitis, muscular dystrophy and, less frequently now in most countries, empyema or surgical treatment for tuberculosis. When severe, these conditions may result in inadequate or uneven ventilation, compression of the lung, atelectasis, reduced compliance and a tendency to respiratory infections. The physiological and pathological consequences include arterial hypoxaemia, hypercapnia, pulmonary hypertension causing hypertrophy and dilatation of the right ventricle and finally cardiac failure (pulmonary heart disease).

Spondylosis

Spondylosis or spondylitis, involving the cervical or thoracic vertebrae, may be responsible for referred pain simulating that of coronary heart disease, as may any condition involving the same sensory pathways. Sometimes pain is felt also in the back, but more infrequently only anteriorly. Pain may occur on exertion or spontaneously during the night or on the day following unusual exertion or posture. Thoracic kyphosis may also be responsible for referred pain which is aggravated by exertion. Skeletal pain is sometimes relieved, at least partially, by nitroglycerin which, in consequence, is of little value as a therapeutic test in the differential diagnosis of pain in the chest.

Ankylosing spondylitis may be associated with aortic regurgitation.

Straight-back syndrome

Absence of the normal dorsal kyphosis, sometimes known as the 'straight-back syndrome', may be accompanied by a parasternal systolic murmur and unusually wide separation of the two components of the second heart sound. This murmur may be accentuatd by external compression of the chest and decreases, often markedly, on deep inspiration.

Rounded configuration of the chest wall

A barrel-shaped chest may be due to an emphysema but is an unreliable sign. Emphysema may occur in its absence or may be severe with a normal-shaped chest. On the other hand, a rounded configuration of the chest wall may be responsible for relative faintness of heart sounds or murmurs owing to the increased distance and the tissues between the heart and stethoscope.

Neuromuscular disorders

There are a number of hereditary neuromuscular disorders associated with degenerative changes, fibrosis or hypertrophy of the myocardium. They are reflected clinically in enlargement of the heart, dysrhythmias, defects of conduction, gallop rhythm, non-specific electrocardiographic abnormalities and cardiac failure. There is no specific treatment but the physician should be aware of the association of heart disease with, in particular, Friedreich's ataxia, pseudohypertrophic muscular dystrophy and myotonia atrophica.

The Marfan syndrome

The Marfan syndrome is an inherited defect of connective tissue and the clinical manifestations include skeletal and cardiovascular abnormalities and, particularly in the present context, dilatation of the thoracic aorta and aortic regurgitation. Other valvar defects and congenital lesions, and also dysrhythmias and defects of conduction, may occur.

The presenting skeletal features often include thinness, tallness, long slender extremities, arachnodactyly, deformities of the chest and spine, hyperextensible joints and deformities of the feet.

Dissecting aneurysm of the aorta may be a fatal complication.

2

Auscultation

'I hear, I hear, with joy I hear'
— Wordsworth.

All students at first find difficulty with auscultation and to some heart sounds and murmurs remain a mystery. However, given sufficient interest, normal hearing, a good stethoscope and an appreciation of underlying mechanisms together with reasonable opportunity to practise, anyone can become sufficiently competent.

The essential requirements are a methodical approach with attention to detail and accurate recording of what is heard. This will usually lead to correct diagnosis.

Recognition of auscultatory phenomena is important, not only for accurate diagnosis but to avoid errors of interpretation and, in particular, the frequent error of suspecting or actually diagnosing heart disease when none is present and thereby engendering anxiety or imposing unwarranted restrictions. The latter may be a greater evil than failure to recognise mild organic disease.

The presence or absence of heart disease can frequently be determined by auscultation and often a reliable assessment of the severity of a valve lesion or of some types of congenital heart defect can be made. However apart from the presence or absence of a gallop rhythm no reliable assessment of the severity of cardiac failure can be obtained from auscultation of the heart.

Beginners, of course, find difficulty from lack of experience and there is a danger that errors which are uncorrected at this stage will be perpetuated. However, difficulty is often largely due to lack of good technique and of appreciation that there is a rational and usually simple explanation for all that can be heard.

The adoption of a diagrammatic record of the auscultatory findings is recommended as a stimulus to accuracy, to save time, and to give an independent observer a clear idea of exactly what has been heard (Fig. 8).

More advanced students are often more familiar with what they have been told or read than with bedside observation and tend to find physical signs which they consider 'ought' to be present rather than to record what can actually be heard. Objectivity is essential and the physician should record what

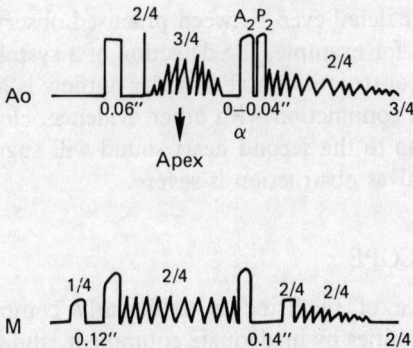

Fig. 8 The auscultatory diagram. In written form this would read: There is a moderate aortic systolic ejection click heard 0.06 s after the first sound, followed by a loud aortic systolic ejection murmur conducted to the apex. The second sound is normally split varying from single on expiration to 0.04 s on inspiration and is followed by a moderate intensity, early diastolic murmur extending threequarters of the way through diastole. There is a soft fourth sound 0.12 s before the first sound, a moderate intensity, mitral regurgitant (pansystolic) murmur, a moderate third sound 0.14 s after aortic closure, followed by a moderate intensity, mitral mid-diastolic murmur extending halfway through diastole.

has actually been detected and never what he thinks ought to have been heard, based on a preconceived idea of the diagnosis. Conversely, any findings which do not apparently 'fit' with the remaining examination or with other investigations such as echocardiography or cardiac catheterisation must not be discarded without careful reappraisal.

Older physicians often find difficulty because they were trained before the days of modern precision which is due to the more accurate analysis of valve movement and time intervals made possible by echocardiographic phonocardiographic studies, and the stimulus to accuracy provided by the information obtained at cardiac catheterisation and cardiac surgery.

Sometimes seemingly undue attention is given by specialists to what might be determined the minutiae of auscultation which may appear to be of academic interest rather than practical value, and at the bedside there may be a difference of opinion over detail even between practised observers. On the other hand, for example, the detection of a systolic click may signify that obstruction to ventricular outflow is at valve level or, taken in conjunction with other evidence, closeness of an opening snap to the second heart sound will suggest that the degree of valvar obstruction is severe.

STETHOSCOPE

The practice of medicine is sufficiently complex without adding difficulties by inadequate equipment, and a small extra financial outlay will pay good dividends over the years.

Man mainly hears, as he sees, what he knows and the most important part of the hearing apparatus is the sophisticated computer which lies between the ear pieces of the stethoscope. However, it is surprising to find that some physicians, if few students, still possess a stethoscope with only a bell chest piece. Anyone having doubts as to the value of the diaphragm will soon have them removed by comparing the relative intensity of a high pitched murmur with both types of chest piece. The best example is the familiar early diastolic murmur of aortic regurgitation. Such a murmur is always better heard with a diaphragm and, if faint, may not be audible at all with a bell. Similarly, the low pitched, rumbling, apical diastolic murmur, which is characteristic of mitral stenosis, may be more readily heard with a bell and missed altogether with a diaphragm.

The modern stethoscope is a precision instrument which has been carefully designed to give the best acoustic performance. The student buying his first stethoscope is confronted with a bewildering range of designs and prices. There are a number of similarities between buying a stethoscope and buying a car and in both cases the final choice depends on individual preference. Nevertheless, there are some fundamental physical principles which govern the correct design *and use* of a stethoscope.

Transmission of sound is damped by air and consequently the length of tubing is important — the shorter the better. A length of 25–30 cm (10–12 inches) is optimal, but many stethoscopes have much longer tubing. In these it is usually possible to trim the excess length of tubing from the end nearest the chest piece. For the same reason the internal volume of the system should be kept as small as is practicable and tubing should have an internal diameter of about 0.3 cm (0.125 inches). The wall of the tubing should be flexible but sufficiently thick to suppress outside noise. Although there are theoretical advantages in having separate tubes connecting the chest piece with the ear pieces, this is at the expense of an increase in internal volume of the system and for practical purposes the single tube connected by a Y piece to the ear piece tubes which has been adopted by many manufacturers, holds no disadvantages and is less bulky. As the stethoscope tubing will usually wear out long before the rest of the instrument, it is an advantage to be able to replace this. In some modern designs the tubing is moulded to the ear piece tubes and cannot be replaced separately.

There must be no air leaks from the system or the frequency response may be drastically altered. Ear pieces must therefore fit snugly and comfortably and their optimal size and shape must be determined by the individual. Some manufacturers provide interchangeable ear pieces of different sizes and shapes. For a snug and comfortable fit the forward angulation of the ear piece tubes and the pressure exerted by the ear pieces should be adjustable. The tension can usually be adjusted by gently bending the spring connection between the ear piece tubes and the angulation varied either by rotation of the individual ear piece tubes in the moulded design of stethoscope or by the use of a hinged spring connection between the two ear pieces. If the latter is used it is important that it is not loose and liable to rattle. When the bell is being used airtight application of the chest piece to the patient's skin must be possible without undue pressure. The larger the area covered the better the volume of sound. However if the bell is too large in a patient with a bony chest, a complete seal around the edges will not be obtained without using moderate pressure. This may stretch the skin thus converting it into a diaphragm and modifying what can be heard. In fact, varying the pressure which is applied by the chest piece to the skin is a useful means of enhancing various sounds and murmurs and full advantage of this should be taken. To facilitate an airtight fit, some manufacturers use a thin rim of rubber around the rim of the bell.

To achieve good attenuation of the loud low frequency components of the heart sounds and murmurs and allow selective transmission of the high frequency components, the diaphragm type chest piece needs to be flat. The diaphragm itself serves to prevent an air leak from the system and the skin from obliterating the shallow cavity of the diaphragm. Provided these two conditions are met the frequency response of the stethoscope is not materially affected if the diaphragm itself is removed completely. Conversely the diaphragm should not be too thick to allow free transmission of sound from the chest wall into the stethoscope.

It is in design of the chest piece that the greatest variation occurs between different models of stethoscopes as this is the main factor in determining the frequency response of the instrument. The commonest modern design incorporates a single diaphragm and bell, selected by rotating the chest piece around the tubing attachment. Some chest pieces incorporate two different diaphragms and a bell in order to increase the selectivity of frequency response. These instruments however are bulky and heavy and the purchaser needs to be satisfied that the advantages, if any, of the system are sufficient to justify this. A stethoscope spends a lot of its time around the user's neck and a heavy unwieldy instrument can be a serious disadvantage. However some of the 'lightweight' stethoscopes are of flimsy design with tubing of inadequate thickness.

In a recent evaluation by one of us (R.G.G.) in conjunction with an acoustic physicist, the objectively measured frequency responses of most of the popular modern stethoscopes incorporating a single diaphragm and bell varied so little as to be most unlikely to be detected by even a trained observer. Despite this, physicians have very firmly held opinions as to the advantages and disadvantages of various models of stethoscope, a situation which again has its parallel in the choice of a car!

The main criticism of this evaluated group of stethoscopes is an inadequate attenuation of low frequencies when using the diaphragm. The produces a relatively loud acoustic response but results in some of the important high-frequency information being drowned by the much louder low-frequency components. It is important to realise that the stethoscope which produces the loudest noise is not necessarily the best. Nevertheless this type of stethoscope offers the student a modern, usually well constructed, stethoscope, quite satisfactory for general use. The prices vary by several pounds and do not necessarily reflect superiority. In the more traditional and generally more expensive group of stethoscopes improved high-frequency response was noted in some but this was quite variable. However construction on the whole was more robust, using heavier metal and rubber rather than the modern instruments' alloy and plastic. The bulky multiple-headed stethoscopes appeared to have no advantage over the simpler single diaphragm and bell models.

Of all the stethoscopes tested only one, the Rappaport-Sprague stethoscope was found to have a markedly superior high-frequency response but its price of more than £80 places it well out of the reach of the average student.

A stethoscope lasts a very long time and will be used more frequency than any other instrument the student or physician purchases. As with a car, familiarity with a particular model often more than compensates for minor defects in it and for this reason the prospective purchaser should try to obtain the instrument on at least a week's approval before making a final decision.

TECHNIQUE OF AUSCULTATION

Practice tends to make perfect, but everyone will agree that all the practice in the world will not necessarily make a good musician, golfer or physician. Nevertheless, skill with auscultation does come with practice and every beginner will be pleasantly surprised at how much can be heard when something has been pointed out and the lesson has been learned of *listening methodically to one thing at a time*. Auscultation should always be deliberate and never casual.

It is not necessary to be musically inclined to acquire skill in auscultation. A convenient simile is provided by the fact that, with practice in listening to a large orchestra, different instruments such as an oboe may be distinguished, whereas initially only an overall impression of sound will be appreciated. Likewise with auscultation, experience will bring appreciation of an added sound or high-pitched murmur that has been missed by the relatively inexperienced or casual observer. However it must be said that the student who is tone deaf and lacking in any sense of rhythm may be in difficulties!

It is best to begin by concentrating on the *normal heart sounds* and trying to distinguish both components.

The mitral component of the first heart sound is best heard at the apex and the tricuspid component at the lower left sternal border.

The aortic component of the second sound is usually best heard to the right of the upper sternal border, or over it, and the pulmonary component to the left of the upper sternal border.

The component of the second heart sound that can be heard at the apex is usually derived from the aortic valve, the pulmonary component only being audible at the apex in cases of pulmonary hypertension or sometimes when wide splitting of the second heart sound, as in bundle branch block, makes the separation of the two components very distinct.

After this it should be determined whether or not *additional sounds* are present and their positions in the cardiac cycle in relation to the two main sounds, preferably by indicating the interval in seconds after or before the nearest major heart sound.

Then, forgetting about sounds, attention should be paid to *murmurs*, first in systole, that is between the first and second heart sounds, and then in diastole, that is between the second and first sounds.

It is a good plan, having detected the presence of a murmur and its position of maximum intensity, gradually to 'edge' the stethoscope out in each direction to note its 'propagation' or 'conduction'. In some cases this procedure greatly facilitates diagnosis. For example, if a systolic murmur is loudest at the left mid or lower sternal border and can be traced best up and to the right, perhaps into the neck over the carotid artery, it is probably arising from the outflow tract of the left ventricle. If an apical systolic murmur is best conducted to the axilla, or beyond to the left lung base, it is more likely to be arising from the mitral value and indicate mitral regurgitation.

In general, however, a murmur is also 'conducted' in proportion to its intensity and too much attention should not be paid to propagation.

Cardiac enlargement is another important factor. For example, with dilatation of the right ventricle, a tricuspid systolic murmur may be well heard at the apex.

The origin of the murmur may sometimes be determined by the accurate localisation of the corresponding thrill.

Full advantage should be taken of simple manoeuvres which may facilitate auscultation and hence accurate interpretation. These include posture, respiration, exercise, the Valsalva manoeuvre and occasionally the administration of an appropriate drug to alter systemic arterial resistance.

POSTURE AND RESPIRATION

Posture

In the reclining posture venous return to the heart is increased and this can be further augmented by raising the legs. Most murmurs and gallop rhythms are louder in the lying position.

Mitral murmurs are best heard if the patient is turned on to the left side, bringing the apex of the heart closer to the chest wall. Mitral thrills are likewise best felt in this position.

An aortic diastolic murmur is best heard with the patient sitting up and leaning forward with the breath held in expiration.

Presystolic and early diastolic gallop rhythms of left heart origin are better heard with the patient supine, often when turned to the left side. Likewise, the associated additional impulse on palpation will be better appreciated in this position. Such added sounds and pulsations may disappear with the patient sitting or standing.

Respiration

Inspiration, by decreasing intrapleural pressure, increases venous return to the right cardiac chambers from the extra-thoracic vessels with consequent prolongation of right ventricular (RV) systole and delay in pulmonary valve closure. At the same time, pulmonary capacity is increased with a resultant delay in venous return to the left atrium and consequent shortening of left ventricular (LV) systole and earlier closure of the aortic valve. As a result, right sided cardiac events are usually louder during inspiration and left sided events a few seconds later.

The effects of respiration are of particular value in regard to the two components of the second sound and to tricuspid murmurs.

Initially, auscultation should be carried out with the patient supine during quiet respiration, then, after instruction on how to breathe, whilst taking a long, slow breath, and then stopping *without* performing a Valsalva manoeuvre, and finally breathing out and holding the breath in full expiration. If the patient takes too deep and too rapid a breath the glottis may be closed at the end of inspiration, causing a sharp increase in intrathoracic pressure (the Valsalva manoeuvre), thereby annulling the desired effect of inspiration. For this reason, alternatively the patient may be asked simply to take deep slow breaths in and out without holding the breath at any stage.

In health, both components of the second sound can usually be distinguished at the end of deep inspiration, but fuse into an apparently single sound during expiration. This is *normal splitting*. Abnormally wide splitting occurs in right bundle branch block or in conditions producing prolongation of right ventricular systole and delay in pulmonary valve closure such as pulmonary stenosis or right ventricular dysfunction. However, the mode of splitting is still normal in that it is widest on inspiration. If the splitting is wide enough the second sound may still be audibly split on expiration but becoming much more widely split on inspiration. Occasionally separation of the two components occurs during expiration owing to prolongation of *left* ventricular systole and delay in *aortic* valve closure. This *reversed splitting* ('*paradoxical*' *splitting*) is a feature of left bundle branch block, severe aortic stenosis, large patent ductus arteriosus and left ventricular dysfunction from coronary heart disease and hypertension.

Fixed splitting is the characteristic feature of an atrial septal defect. The separation of the two components is 'fixed' and uninfluenced by respiration. This is because the atrial septal defect allows free transmission of the pressure changes occurring with respiration in the right atrium to the left atrium. Splitting of the second sound is discussed in greater detail on p. 76.

The systolic ejection click of pulmonary valve stenosis of more than a mild degree is loudest on expiration and becomes softer or even disappears during inspiration. This feature is a guide to the severity of the stenosis (p. 72).

Right sided gallop rhythms are usually best heard on inspiration and left sided gallop rhythms on expiration.

Left heart murmurs are best heard in expiration, partly because there is less lung to dampen conduction between the heart and the chest wall and partly because blood flow through the left heart is greatest in expiration. Blood is held up in the lungs during inspiration, due to their expansion and the increased negative intrathoracic pressure. On the other hand, the intensity of right heart murmurs is often increased by inspiration when there is an increase in the degree of negative pressure in the thorax and consequently increased venous return to the right side of the heart. Tricuspid systolic and diatolic murmurs are frequently missed through failure to listen as a routine during deep inspiration.

When cardiac failure is present the heart may be maximally loaded even in expiration and consequently no inspiratory increase in the murmur is noted.

Exercise

Exercise is occasionally of value in bringing out a doubtful murmur, for example, a faint apical diastolic murmur from mitral stenosis by increasing blood flow. In the outpatient department the heart rate can be conveniently increased by 'running on the spot' with knees raised high, and in the ward by repeatedly sitting up to touch the toes and lying back.

Valsalva manoeuvre

In the Valsalva manoeuvre the subject is asked to carry out forced expiration against a closed glottis. This has the effect of decreasing venous return to the heart. On releasing the breath there is an *immediate* increase in right sided cardiac filling, which thus facilitates recognition of right sided events.

Drugs

The inhalation of amyl nitrite, which lowers the systemic vascular resistance, increases the intensity of left sided murmurs. Likewise, the administration of phenylephrine, which raises the systemic vascular resistance, has the opposite effect.

On occasion these may be useful bedside tests when differentiation is difficult, but in practice they are rarely used.

AREAS OF AUSCULTATION

A word must be said about the 'conventional' areas of auscultation because, especially in patients with heart disease, they are often inaccurate, misleading and reflect outdated concepts.

The aortic area does *not* lie over the aortic valve and in any case an aortic systolic murmur is often loudest over the sternum, at the left sternal border or at the apex. An aortic diastolic murmur is *usually* loudest at the left sternal border. In aortic stenosis the pulmonary component of the second heart sound may alone be audible in the aortic area. In pulmonary stenosis the aortic component of the second sound may alone be audible in the pulmonary area.

In mitral disease the heart is usually enlarged and mitral murmurs or an important third heart sound are often loudest well to the left of the conventional mitral area. On the other hand, the mitral opening snap is often best heard close to the left sternal border. A systolic murmur due to mitral regurgitation from prolapse of the posterior leaflet of the mitral valve may be loudest in the aortic area. A systolic murmur, loudest in the mitral area, may derive from the tricuspid or aortic valves.

When the right heart is enlarged tricuspid murmurs may be heard best, or only heard, well to the left of the conventional tricuspid area and sometimes at the apex or in the epigastrium.

Errors of interpretation are not infrequently made through adherence to these conventional areas. It would be more accurate to use the terms aortic, pulmonary, left atrial, right atrial, left ventricular and right ventricular areas for the regions of the chest wall overlying these chambers. However, it is best to listen over the entire praecordium, to note the precise region in which sounds or murmurs can be heard and where they are loudest, and to draw conclusions from consideration of all the available data. Auscultation must to some extent be interpretative and the diagrammatic representation of the auscultatory findings (Fig. 8) should be labelled according to the valve of origin of the findings, not the auscultatory area where they have been heard. If the latter is unusual it may be indicated by an additional annotation.

THE DISCIPLINE OF AUSCULTATION

> *'And sanctifying by such discipline*
> *Both pain and fear — until we recognise*
> *A grandeur in the beatings of the heart.'*
> — Wordsworth.

Sounds

Are both heart sounds present and, if so, is each normal?

If not, is the *first sound* louder or weaker than normal (or absent)? Can both components be identified?

Is the *second sound* louder or weaker than normal (or absent)?

Does the second sound split normally on inspiration?

Is the splitting reversed, that is, widest on expiration?

Are there more than two heart sounds?

If so, is the *extra sound* in systole or in diastole? Is it nearer the first or the second sound? By what interval? What is its quality? Does it vary with respiration?

Is either sound preceded or followed by a murmur?

Murmurs

If a murmur is heard there should follow a similar mental catechism.

Over what area is it audible and where is it loudest?

In which direction is it next loudest or 'conducted', and how far from the position of maximum intensity can it be heard?

What are its time relationships to the heart sounds? Duration can be graded as short, medium and long.

Is it *systolic* or *diastolic*?

If systolic, does it occur in early, mid or late systole, or is it pansystolic?

If diastolic, is it early, that is immediately following the second sound, or 'mid', that is after an appreciable gap from the second sound or late, that is presystolic?

As will become clear when dealing with individual defects and diseases, each of these features has a particular significance in diagnosis.

An attempt at grading the intensity and describing the qualities of a murmur should always be made. It does not matter how many grades are used by different observers so long as the standard is stated. This can be expressed as a fraction.

If, for example, a systolic murmur is recorded as grade 3/6 intensity, this signifies that the maximal number of grades recognised by the observer is 6, so that the faintest is grade 1, the loudest likely to be heard is grade 6 and the murmur in question is a moderately loud one. Grade 6 should be reserved for the rare occasion when a murmur is so loud that it can be heard without placing the stethoscope on the chest wall.

Grading by auscultation can only be approximate and variable because subjective. However, the three grades, faint, moderately loud and very loud, sometimes used are not sufficient if changes over a period are to be recorded.

As regards quality it would be helpful if agreement could be reached over adjectives, and preferably their number should be restricted.

It is suggested that the terms *blowing*, *harsh* or *rumbling*, and *high* or *low* pitched will cover most types or murmur. Additional terms are sometimes needed to describe unusual murmurs such as whistling, musical, raucous or the so-called 'seagull' murmur.

Murmurs often vary from day-to-day and hour-to-hour, depending on changes in cardiac output and blood flow. These in turn are influenced by rest, emotion, temperature, heart rate and other factors such as anaemia.

GENESIS OF HEART SOUNDS AND MURMURS

Over the years there has been a large amount of speculation and assumption as to the origin of heart sounds and murmurs. Heart sounds have been variously ascribed to vibrations set up by abrupt changes in the velocity of the blood stream, for example by valve closure suddenly arresting or reversing the movement of blood, to the coaptation of the valve cusps to vibrations of the ventricular wall and to billowing of the valve leaflets and tension on the chordae tendineae. As a result of echocardiographic and phonocardiographic studies coupled with careful examination of the blood flow, force of ventricular contraction and the pressure and sound waves generated within the cardiac chambers and the use of high speed motion pictures of valves mounted in a hydraulic model of the cardiovascular system, a large amount of evidence has accrued to indicate that vibrations set up in the heart valves immediately *after* closure are responsible for the production of heart sounds.

The term *turbulence* has long been used to explain the production of heart murmurs. Later, opinion favoured as an explanation, the creation of vortices in the wake of an obstruction or irregularity in much the same way as the Aeolian harp used by the ancients produced its tones. This view was based on the inability to demonstrate in the cardiovascular system the presence of those conditions which had been shown to be necessary to produce true turbulence when studying flow in smooth straight pipes. With the development of more refined techniques for the detection of turbulence and the ability to use these techniques in the human cardiovascular system, it has now been shown that turbulence does indeed occur in the human circulation and is very likely responsible for the production of ejection murmurs and possibly of regurgitant murmurs. Furthermore these techniques have failed to demonstrate any evidence of periodic vortex shedding (Aeolian tones) as a mechanism for the genesis of heart murmurs.

It is postulated that the fluctuating velocities and pressures due to the turbulence set up local vibrations in the vessel wall which are then transmitted to the surface of the chest. Intracardiac phonocardiography has shown that murmurs are conducted in the direction of the flow of blood through the orifice responsible for the murmur and are not heard upstream from it. This suggests that very little conduction of sound occurs through the blood by compression waves. On the other hand vibrations set up, for example, in the wall of the aorta close to a stenosed aortic valve are often well transmitted downstream along the wall of the vessel so that the murmur is well heard in the carotid or sometimes even the brachial arteries.

PHONOCARDIOGRAPHY

Phonocardiography is the graphic registration of heart sounds and murmurs. A specially designed microphone is placed on the chest wall and the vibrations produced by the heart are picked up, amplified, filtered and recorded.

The microphone has the property of converting sounds or pressure waves into electric currents and responds fairly uniformly over the range of frequencies required in phonocardiography.

Phonocardiography has brought precision to auscultation and, having laid the basis for the correct appreciation of auscultatory findings, is now principally of use as a reference for accurate timing of events in cases of dispute, for teaching and research, and to provide a visual record, as may be necessary for publication.

Heart sounds and murmurs are timed against an electrocardiogram. An external carotid arterial tracing, a jugular phlebogram or an apex displacement cardiogram or, on occasion, the pressure tracings from a cardiac catheter are also used as additional sources of reference. In some cases great precision may be obtained by intracardiac phonocardiography using a phonocatheter which has the sound transducer at its tip. For research purposes amplitude-calibrated phonocardiography and frequency spectrum analysis provide more detailed information regarding the intensity and quality of heart sounds and murmurs.

High quality phonocardiography demands good apparatus, good technical assistance and, above all, the personal attention of a physician with plenty of time and patience and with knowledge of each patient and the points to be determined. It is thus a highly subjective technique and inappropriate microphone placement, filter selection or gain adjustment may drastically influence the interpretation of the phonocardiogram. A misconception not infrequently held by students is that the phonocardiograph is able to record sounds and murmurs which the auscultator is unable to detect. With the possible exception of a soft third or fourth heart sound, this is completely untrue. On the contrary an elusive soft, high frequency, aortic diastolic murmur which has been detected by an experienced auscultator may be difficult or impossible to detect on the phonocardiogram.

Phonocardiography is no substitute for auscultation.

ECHOCARDIOGRAPHY

The most important non-invasive diagnostic tool to be developed in cardiology in recent years is the technique of echocardiography. This is a method of producing visual images of anatomical structures of the heart by the use of very high frequency sound waves of approximately 100 times higher frequency than the upper limit of audible sound. It employs the same principles as sonar, the echo-sounding equipment developed for detecting submarines, shoals of fish and assessing the depth of the sea bed. A beam of high-frequency sound waves is directed into the heart from a transducer held in contact with the chest wall. When the ultrasonic wave strikes a boundary between tissues of different densities part of the wave is reflected back to the surface and is detected by the transducer. In order to avoid confusion between the outgoing and reflected signals the beam of ultrasound is split up into a series of rapid pulses so that the time between each pulse allows for the return of the echo to the transducer. The time taken for each pulse of ultrasound to return to the transducer is measured and from this the distance of the reflecting boundary from the transducer can be determined. Each pulse produces a new set of measurements and the pulses are so frequent that even the fastest moving structures in the heart can be detected. The echo signals are processed electronically to remove unwanted noise and to enhance the fainter echoes arising from structures more distant from the transducer. The resultant echo signals are projected from a specially designed oscilloscope onto a moving strip of photographic paper. By this means a continuous record the M-mode echocardiogram, is obtained of the echoes from structures lying in the path of the beam from the transducer. As the structures giving rise to the echoes move towards and away from the transducer, this movement is indicated by an upward and downward movement respectively on the echocardiogram. Thus in the case of examination of the mitral valve for example, with the transducer applied to the anterior chest near the sternal border, forward movement of a mitral valve leaflet is indicated by an upward movement of its corresponding echo tracing on the echocardiogram.

For greater detail of how this process is achieved the reader should refer to one of the text books devoted to the subject of echocardiography. It is however important to realise that with this type of display only structures lying in the path of the beam will be recorded. The direction of the beam of ultrasound to pick up the various structures one wishes to examine necessitates considerable training and experience together with a knowledge of the anatomy of the underlying structures being examined and a familiarity with their echocardiographic appearance. In this respect the echocardiogram is thus as subjective as the interpretation of auscultatory findings.

If the direction of the beam is rotated, different areas of the heart will come to lie in the path of the beam. By achieving a rapid sweep of the beam across as wide an area of the heart as possible a two-dimensional image of the heart can be built up. This may be achieved by using a special type of echo probe which contains several transducers whose beams are made to scan a roughly triangular area beneath the transducer, with the apex of the triangle being nearest to the transducer. Alternatively a large number of transducers may be mounted side by side, the so-called 'phased-array'. The resultant image bears much more resemblance anatomically to a two-dimensional cross-section of the heart and this type of display is known as a real-time two-dimensional (2-D) echocardiogram. As with the M-mode display, movement can be seen as it occurs but because of the greater similarity to the actual underlying anatomy it is easier for the less experienced observer to relate the movement of the structures seen on this type of display to the events taking place in the cardiac cycle.

Echocardiography can be combined with phonocardiography and/or an apex cardiogram and the superimposition of phonocardiogram, electrocardiogram and an M-mode echocardiogram provides an excellent means of studying the precise timing of movements of the heart valves and their relationship to the sounds and murmurs being produced. The application of this technique has greatly enhanced our present knowledge of the origin of heart sounds and murmurs.

While offering a number of advantages, the 2-D real-time echocardiogram requires even more experience and skill on the part of the operator to produce good quality images than does the M-mode echocardiogram. Furthermore the equipment for this type of display is still very expensive and is thus at the moment unlikely to be found outside of the larger hospitals with specialised cardiological departments.

USES OF ECHOCARDIOGRAPHY

As with phonocardiography, *echocardiography is not a substitute for careful auscultation and clinical examination*. In some situations it has the capability of producing an anatomically precise diagnosis, to a greater degree than is possible by clinical examination and auscultation. In other situations, notably in valvular heart disease, the experienced auscultator can not only arrive at the correct diagnosis at least as often as the echocardiographer, but also obtain a more reliable estimate of the severity of the condition from clinical examination than is possible with the echocardiogram. It is therefore useful for the student of cardiology to have a working knowledge of the advantages and limitations of echocardiography and to be to some extent selective when requesting an echocardiogram. Likewise it behoves the echocardiographer not to allow enthusiasm for this unquestionably exciting and rapidly advancing science to lead to over-interpretation of the echocardiographic findings.

Congenital heart disease

It is in this field, particularly since the advent of high resolution 2-D echocardiography that the greatest contributions have been made to the diagnostic accuracy. Indeed in some conditions such as atrial septal defect careful clinical examination supplemented by 2-D echocardiography has led to a significant reduction in the number of patients requiring cardiac catheterisation as a prerequisite to surgical repair of the defect. In an infant with complex cyanotic congenital heart disease, auscultation frequently fails to provide a definitive diagnosis. Echocardiography on the other hand, if not producing the complete diagnosis will often provide extremely useful information of the anatomical abnormalities present to serve as a guide to the operator during subsequent cardiac catheterisation. With increasing technological refinement the anatomical detail provided by the echocardiogram is becoming increasingly greater but the ability to assess and particularly to quantitate physiological functions is rather less reliable.

Contrast echocardiography, employing the ability of ultrasound to detect micro-bubbles in fluid injected into the circulation is often useful to detect an abnormal communication between two chambers such as a ventricular septal defect. However it is not able to quantitate the degree of shunting of blood or the direction of the shunt. For instance, bubbles in fluid injected into the peripheral vein of a child with a ventricular septal defect can pass from right ventricle to left ventricle even in the presence of a large left to right shunt. New techniques employing the Doppler principle, capable of measuring the amount and direction of blood flow may with further refinement provide the physiological information which is at present somewhat lacking in the echocardiogram.

Valvular heart disease

Echocardiography particularly when combined with phonocardiography enables identification and timing of the movement of the heart valves with great precision (Fig. 9). It can also identify abnormalities of valve movement and anatomical irregularities such as thickening and calcification of a valve, abnormalities of movement of a prosthetic heart valve or the presence of vegetations due to infective endocarditis. The mitral and aortic valves are usually easily examined by M-mode echocardiography but the pulmonary and tricuspid valves may be more difficult or impossible to visualise in some subjects. Even very mild *mitral stenosis* producing minimal auscultatory

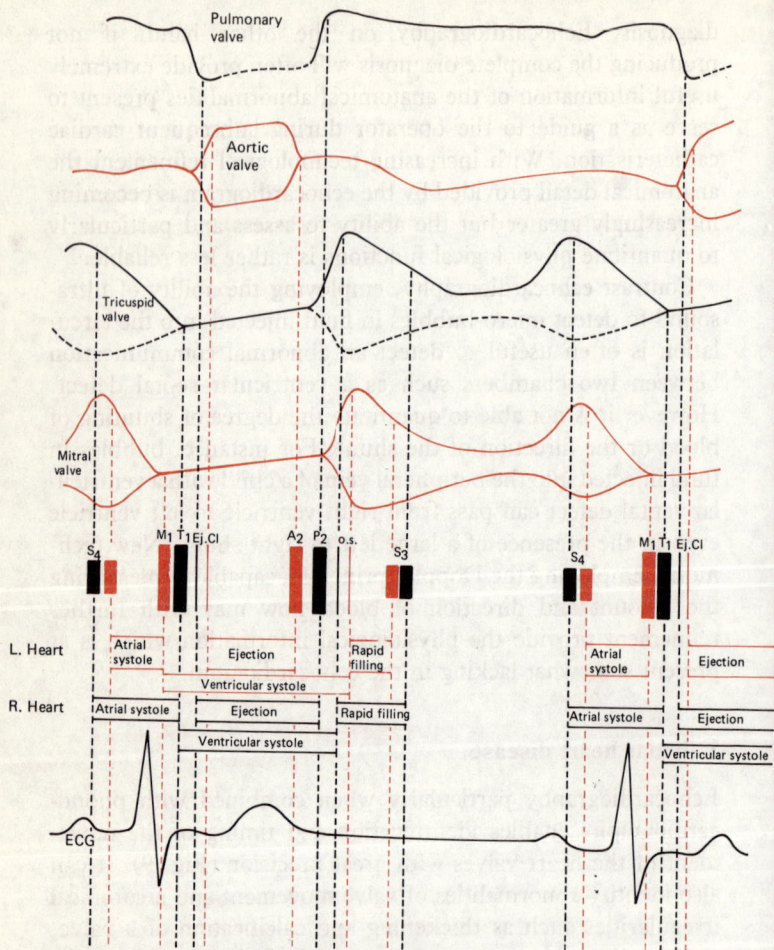

Fig. 9 Heart sounds and the echocardiogram. This is a composite diagram to illustrate the relationship of the various heart sounds to the events in the cardiac cycle and the corresponding movement of the heart valves as recorded in the M-mode echocardiogram. In reality all four heart valves are never visible in the same echocardiogram. The broken lines in the pulmonary and tricuspid valve tracings indicate that these parts of the valve movements are not usually visible.

signs is readily detectable by echocardiography and this feature is useful in differentiating between the mitral diastolic murmur of minimal mitral stenosis and that due to the presence of aortic regurgitation (the Austin-Flint murmur). The severity of mitral stenosis is however often over-estimated by echocardiography if only the pattern of movement of the mitral valve leaflets on the M-mode echocardiogram is used. Even using more sophisticated computer-aided study of the filling pattern of the left ventricle in the M-mode echocardiogram produces an accuracy no greater than that achieved by the experienced auscultator and sometimes falls short of this.

In *aortic stenosis* significant degrees of thickening of the aortic valve especially if accompanied by calcification are usually readily detected by echocardiography but here the quantitation of the severity of the stenosis is less reliable than can be deduced by clinical examination. It is often possible by echocardiography to determine whether the aortic valve has two or three cusps, the presence of dilatation of the aortic root or the presence of a subvalvar or supravalvar as opposed to valvar site of the aortic stenosis.

In *tricuspid stenosis*, provided the tricuspid valve is well visualised, even mild degrees of tricuspid stenosis can be detected by the echocardiograph when, for example, in the presence of a loud mitral opening snap and diastolic murmur the auscultatory evidence of tricuspid stenosis may be difficult to detect.

Provided a good view of the pulmonary valve can be obtained it is possible to detect *pulmonary stenosis* and often with 2-D echocardiography to say whether the stenosis is valvar or infundibular. However auscultation provides a much more accurate estimate of the degree of pulmonary valve stenosis than is possible with echocardiography, provided the atrial and ventricular septa are intact.

Although echocardiography may provide some indirect evidence of the presence of *valvar regurgitation*, such as the vibration seen on the anterior mitral valve leaflet in aortic regurgitation, this evidence is not diagnostic and is of little use in assessing the severity of the regurgitation. This is because the anatomical appearance and mobility of the valve so readily detectable by echocardiography often correlate very poorly with the physiological behaviour of the valve. Clinical examination will usually provide a better guide to the severity of mitral, aortic or tricuspid regurgitation through even here quantitation cannot be as precise as with stenotic lesions.

Assessment of ventricular hypertrophy, dilatation and function.

Left ventricular hypertrophy is readily apparent in the echocardiogram from measurement of the thickness of the posterior wall of left ventricle and of the interventricular septum. Right ventricular hypertrophy is less easy to determine because of the proximity of the anterior wall of the right ventricle to the chest wall. Dilatation of either chamber and of left atrium are readily apparent on M-mode echocardiography and the dimension of the cavity can be measured precisely. Some estimate of right atrial dilatation is obtainable with 2-D echocardiography.

One of the most useful contributions of echocardiography is its ability to provide reliable and quantitative information about *left ventricular function*. Measurement of the maximum and minimum dimensions of the left ventricular cavity in diastole and systole respectively, can be made accurately from a good quality M-mode echocardiogram and hence the ejection fraction of the ventricle obtained. Using computer techniques a large amount of detailed information can be obtained about the pattern of left ventricular contraction. Apart from the detection of reversed splitting of the second heart sound or the presence of a third or fourth sound, auscultation gives no information about left ventricular function.

Used intelligently the combination of accurate auscultation and good quality echocardiography provide a wealth of diagnostic and quantitative information which already has reduced the need for preoperative cardiac catheterisation.

3

Heart sounds

'*A lover's ear will hear*
the lowest sound.'
— Shakespeare.

First heart sound	Mitral component
	Tricuspid component
Second heart sound	Aortic component
	Pulmonary component
Opening snap	Mitral
	Tricuspid
Third heart sound	Right ventricular
	Left ventricular
Fourth heart sound	Right atrial
	Left atrial
Summation gallop	
Ejection click	Aortic
	Pulmonary
Midsystolic click	
Pericardial ('knock')	

FIRST AND SECOND HEART SOUNDS

The conventional explanation for the *first heart sound* has been that it is mainly produced by closure of the mitral and tricuspid valves when ventricular pressure rises above that in the atria. In recent years this view has been challenged and evidence produced which suggests that the first sound actually follows valve closure and is due to vibrations in the closed cusps, chordae, papillary muscles and ventricular walls.

Likewise, the conventional explanation for the *second heart sound* has been that it is due to closure of the aortic and pulmonary valves when ventricular pressure falls below that in the great vessels. Again, recent work has suggested that the second sound actually follows valve closure and is due to vibrations in the closed cusps and adjacent structures.

Whatever the correct explanation, valve closure is the *determining* factor in timing.

Normally the sounds related to mitral and aortic valve closure are louder than those produced in relation to tricuspid and pulmonary valve closure because of greater pressures on the left side of the heart.

Note on terminology

It has been customary to refer to the second heart sound heard in the conventional aortic area as A_2 and that heard in the pulmonary area as P_2 (p. 48). These are convenient abbreviations but, since the second sound consists of two components which it is important to distinguish, A_2 and P_2 should refer to the aortic and pulmonary components respectively regardless of where they are heard.

Heart sounds and murmurs may be difficult to hear on account of:

1. Thickness of the chest wall
2. Increased anteroposterior diameter of the chest
3. Decreased force of cardiac contraction
4. Emphysema
5. Pericardial effusion
6. Factors impairing conduction from the heart to the chest wall

7. Inappropriate stethoscope and chest piece
8. Impaired hearing, especially of high frequency murmurs.

QUALITIES OF THE HEART SOUNDS

The following properties should be noted:

1. Increased intensity
2. Decreased intensity or absence
3. Varying intensity.

Intensity of first heart sound

The conventional explanation has been that the intensity of the first sound in a normal subject is mainly dependent on the postition of the valve leaflets at the onset of ventricular systole and on the force of ventricular contraction. If the valve leaflets were widely separated at the time of onset of ventricular contraction and had a relatively long way to travel in order to shut, the closing sound would be relatively loud because of this, but if the valve was almost closed the closing sound would be relatively faint. All this assumed that the noise of the first sound came from the act of valve closure. Recent work suggests that this is not so and that the first sound arises from vibrations in the mitral and tricuspid valves immediately after closure (see Fig. 9). It is suggested that the most important factor in determining the intensity of the first sound is the rate of change of ventricular pressure at the time of valve closure. The higher this rate the louder will be the vibrations set up immediately after closure. The idea that the intensity of the first sound depends on how widely the valve leaflets are separated at the time of onset of ventricular contraction is however still valid. If the valve is being held widely open by a raised pressure in the atrium immediately before ventricular contraction commences then in order to close the valve the pressure in the ventricle will have had to rise higher than would have been necessary to close a valve which was almost shut, with a lower pressure in the atrium. Because of this the rate of change of ventricular pressure at the time of valve closure will be higher in the case of a valve that was wide open and thus the vibrations set up in the valve immediately after closure will be greater. The valve leaflets will tend to be far apart if ventricular filling is prolonged, as from valvar stenosis or increased blood flow, or if the A–V conduction time is short. Pathological changes causing thickening or rigidity of the valve leaflets are also likely to be important as these cause an increased high frequency component of the vibrations following valve closure which are more readily appreciated by the human ear than the lower frequency components.

The first heart sound tends to be loud with *tachycardia* from any cause such as exercise, emotion, fever or anaemia and with other hyperkinetic circulatory states, such as thyrotoxicosis and pregnancy. The sounds tend to be faint in myocardial infarction, myocardial failure, congestive cardiomyopathy, mitral regurgitation and hypothyroidism.

In *mitral stenosis* the first sound is characteristically loud and slapping, providing the cusps are still mobile. This is probably partly related to the greater rate of change of left ventricular pressure at the moment of mitral valve closure for reasons discussed above and to the higher frequency of the first sound due to the thickening of the valve which occurs in mitral stenosis. A further factor in patients with pulmonary hypertension accompanying mitral stenosis may be the accentuation of the tricuspid component of the first sound.

In *mitral regurgitation* the leaflets may not come together at all, from structural defects or from widening of the valve ring, or they may do so imperfectly. Also, due to the double exit for blood from the left ventricle, the rate of rise of pressure in the ventricle is less. Consequently the first heart sound may be absent or weak.

The intensity of the first sound tends to bear an inverse ratio to the *A–V conduction time* as reflected in the P–R interval of the electrocardiogram, that is, the shorter the P–R interval the louder the sound.

Similarly, *variation in intensity* of the first sound will be present if there is dissociation between atrial and ventricular contraction such as may result from complete heart block, atrial flutter and ventricular tachycardia, when atria and ventricles beat at different rates. The varying intensity of the first heart sound in A–V block may be related to different rates of rise of pressure in the left ventricle at the time of valve closure (see above).

The audible first heart sound is mainly related to mitral valve closure but it is sometimes possible to distinguish increased intensity of the tricuspid component. This will occur in tricuspid stenosis for the same reasons as in mitral stenosis, and in atrial septal defect, where the increased rate of rise of right ventricular pressure consequent upon the increased volume of blood entering it, is probably responsible.

Intensity of the second heart sound

Normally in adults A_2 is louder than P_2 because the diastolic pressure in the aorta exceeds that in the pulmonary artery.

In children, P_2 may be as loud or louder because the pulmonary artery is relatively large and nearer to the chest wall.

Either component may be loud, normal, diminished or absent, depending on intra-arterial pressure and valve movement, and on dilatation of the main vessel together with its proximity to the chest wall and its elasticity which facilitates valve closure.

Increased intensity of the second sound (S_2) at the base of the heart may be due to systemic or pulmonary hypertension. The relationship is not invariable and other factors influence intensity.

A_2 is by no means always loud even in severe systemic hypertension and loudness may be solely due to aortic atherosclerosis. In some cases of severe pulmonary hypertension from mitral stenosis, P_2 may not be loud, possibly from decreased blood flow. Thinness of the chest wall and dilatation of the pulmonary artery are other factors which may increase intensity.

When pulmonary regurgitation is due to severe pulmonary hypertension with normal cusps, P_2 in such cases tends to be loud, but in pulmonary regurgitation from other causes such as cardiac surgery, P_2 may be soft or absent.

Decreased intensity or absence of A_2 or P_2 may result from deficient closure of the semilunar valves.

The *aortic component* may be weak or absent in aortic stenosis or regurgitation, and in such cases S_2 in the pulmonary area, which normally is finely split since closure of both valves can be heard here, will be single. If the *pulmonary component* is loud from pulmonary hypertension in such cases of aortic valvar disease it may also be heard to the right of the sternum.

The pulmonary component is usually weak or absent in pulmonary stenosis, so that S_2 may appear single and derives from the aortic component.

PHYSIOLOGICAL THIRD AND FOURTH HEART SOUNDS

A *third heart sound* may be audible early in diastole, that is shortly after the second sound and during the phase of rapid ventricular filling. It can often be heard in healthy young people.

A *fourth heart sound* late in diastole (presystole), that is just before the first sound, can usually be recorded by phonocardiography but is rarely audible.

These two extra sounds are described in the section on gallop rhythm (p. 83).

SPLITTING OF THE FIRST HEART SOUND

A large amount has been written and a number of contradictory theories advanced as to the composition and origin of the first heart sound. As many as four components have been described as occurring in phonocardiographic records but for practical purposes, on auscultation two principal components may be heard. Whatever the explanation of the mechanism of production of the first sound, it has now been established by combined phono-and echocardiographic recordings that these two components correspond very precisely in timing to the closure of the mitral and tricuspid valves respectively (see Fig. 9). Contraction of the left ventricle normally occurs slightly ahead of that of the right ventricle so that the first component of the first sound is normally associated with mitral valve closure and the second with tricuspid valve closure.

The minimum interval between two components of a heart sound which can be identified by auscultation as distinctly split is around 0.03 s. However the ability to hear a sound as split or not varies considerably with the relative loudness of each component. When the first component is soft and the second is loud, the split is more easily appreciated whereas when the first component is loud and is followed by a relatively soft second component, the split is much more difficult or even impossible to appreciate. As each component of the first heart sound has a duration of around 0.02 s and the normally considerably louder first (mitral) component is separated from the softer second (tricuspid) component by only about 0.03 s the two components frequently merge and are heard as a single sound (Fig. 10).

Normal splitting

This can sometimes be appreciated in healthy subjects by

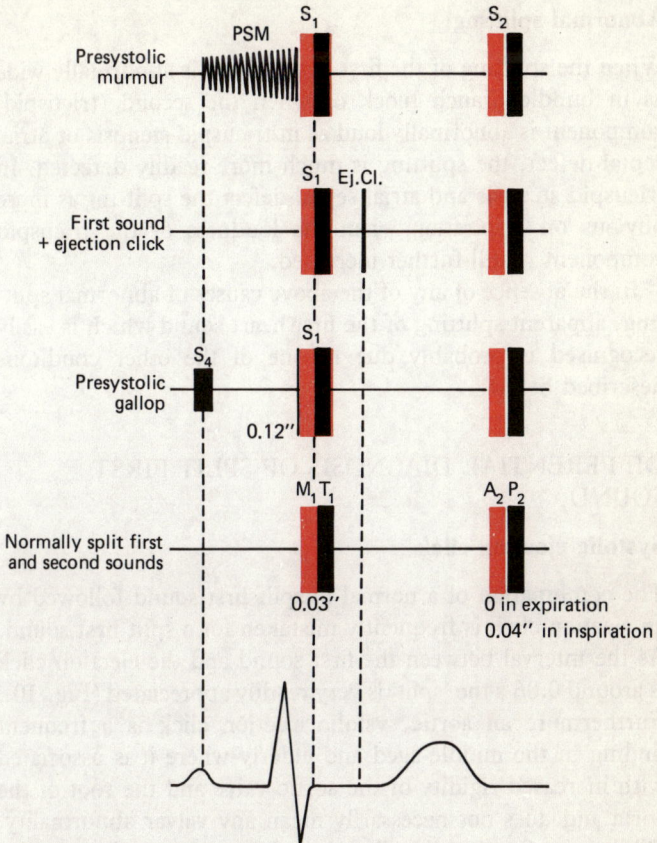

Fig. 10 Differential diagnosis of split first sound. S_1, S_2 and S_4 = first, second and fourth heart sounds; $M_1 T_1$ = mitral and tricuspid components of S_1; A_2P_2 = aortic and pulmonary components of S_2; PSM = presystolic murmur; Ej. Cl. = ejection click.

listening at the lower end of the sternum, which is the position where the stethoscope is nearest to the relatively quiet tricuspid component.

Abnormal splitting

When the splitting of the first heart sound is abnormally wide as in bundle branch block or when the second (tricuspid) component is abnormally loud as in tricuspid stenosis or atrial septal defect, the splitting is much more readily detected. In tricuspid stenosis and atrial septal defect the splitting is more obvious on inspiration when the loudness of the tricuspid component is still further increased.

In the absence of any of the above causes of abnormal splitting, apparent splitting of the first heart sound which is easily recognised is probably due to one of the other conditons described below.

DIFFERENTIAL DIAGNOSIS OF SPLIT FIRST SOUND

Systolic ejection click

The combination of a normal unsplit first sound followed by an ejection click is frequently mistaken for a split first sound. As the interval between the first sound and the ejection click is around 0.06 s the 'split' is very readily appreciated (Fig. 10). Furthermore an aortic systolic ejection click is a frequent finding in the middle-aged and elderly where it is associated with increased rigidity of the aortic valve and the root of the aorta and does not necessarily mean any valvar abnormality. While it is often heard well at the left sternal edge, in the same place as true splitting is best appreciated, the detection of an apparently obvious split first sound at the apex should alert the auscultator to the possibility that the apparent split is in reality a first sound followed by an aortic systolic ejection click. Whereas in true splitting of the first sound the two components are very close together and of somewhat similar quality, the ejection click is usually sharper and higher pitched than the first sound although it may be as loud or even louder. The intensity of an aortic systolic ejection click is usually unaffected by respiration.

A pulmonary systolic ejection click is usually heard best in the pulmonary area but may also be evident at the left sternal edge. When due to pulmonary valve stenosis the ejection click may be loudest on expiration becoming softer or even disappearing on inspiration.

Presystolic gallop rhythm

The presence of a fourth sound followed by a first sound may simulate splitting of the first sound. The fourth sound is however dull and low pitched and usually much softer than the first sound. Furthermore the interval between fourth sound and the first sound is usually much wider, at least 0.12 s (Fig. 10). Some difficulty may however be encountered when the fourth sound is very loud and close to the first sound due to a short P–R interval.

Presystolic murmur

In mitral stenosis with sinus rhythm, atrial systole results in presystolic accentuation of the diastolic murmur at the apex. This murmur becomes louder when blood flow is increased by exercise or tachycardia from any cause. Most often such a murmur is associated with a loud first sound ('closing snap'), an 'opening snap' and a mitral diastolic murmur but, in patients with mild stenosis, only a short presystolic murmur may be present and in such cases there may be difficulty in differentation from splitting of the first heart sound (Fig. 10).

A presystolic murmur becoming louder on inspiration may be heard in tricuspid stenosis and in Ebstein's Anomaly of the tricuspid valve.

SYSTOLIC CLICKS

Early systolic ejection click

This early systolic added sound occurs around 0.06 s after the first sound (Fig. 10). It is relatively high pitched and sharp and is best heard with the diaphragm of the stethoscope. It is sometimes referred to as the opening snap of a semilunar valve.

The ejection click of valve origin has been shown by phono- and echocardiography and by high speed cineangiographic techniques to coincide with the moment at which the respective semilunar valve reaches its fully opened position (Fig. 9) and is probably the result of vibrations set up in the root of the aorta or pulmonary artery respectively by the piston-like action of the valve cusps against the blood within the vessel on opening of the valve and the onset of ejection of blood through it.

Whatever the mechanism, the ejection click provides a precise marker for the onset of ejection and the end of isovolumic contraction of the ventricle. Its recognition is therefore of prime importance in the identification of an ejection systolic murmur.

When associated with stenosis of a semilunar valve the ejection click provides a considerable amount of information.

In *aortic valve stenosis*, observation of an ejection click provides confirmatory evidence that the stenosis is at valve level and not subvalvar or supravalvar and also indicates that the valve is still mobile. The ejection click is lost with heavy calcification of the aortic valve.

A loud systolic ejection click accompanies a congenital *bicuspid aortic valve* even in the absence of any stenosis.

In *pulmonary valve stenosis* the ejection click similarly provides strong evidence that the stenosis is at valve level rather than infundibular. In mild pulmonary valve stenosis the ejection click is present throughout inspiration (Fig. 11a) but in moderate and severe stenosis the click disappears during

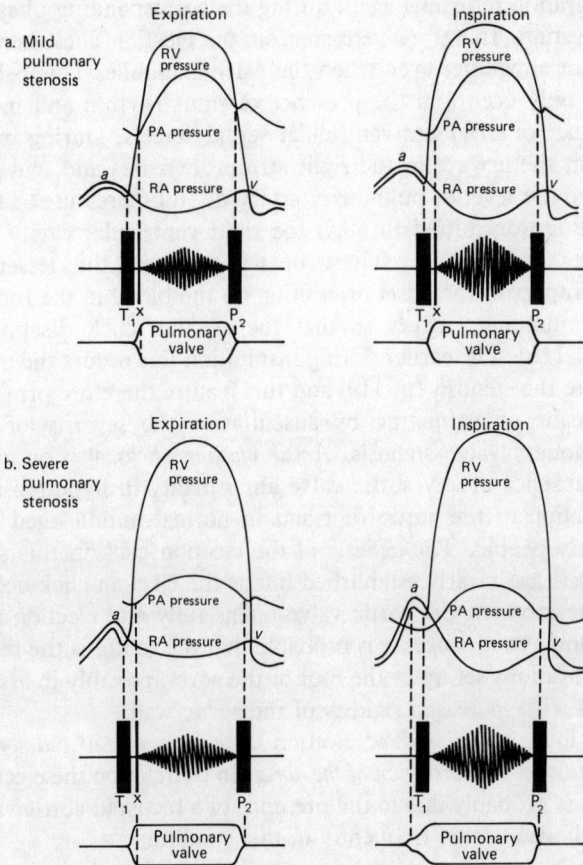

Fig. 11 The behaviour of the pulmonary systolic ejection click with respiration. The relationship of the ejection click (X), the tricuspid component of the first sound (T_1), the pulmonary component of the second sound (P_2) and the pulmonary systolic ejection murmur, to the right atrial (RA), right ventricular (RV) and pulmonary artery (PA) pressures and the opening of the pulmonary valve (illustrated diagrammatically), is shown in full expiration and at the peak of inspiration in (a) mild and (b) severe pulmonary valve stenosis.

inspiration returning again during the corresponding phase of expiration. In very severe stenosis the ejection click may be absent altogether even when the valve is mobile. This behaviour only occurs in the presence of sinus rhythm and in the absence of atrial and ventricular septal defects. During inspiration the *a* wave in the right atrium increases and may rise above the level of pulmonary artery diastolic pressure. The *a* wave is transmitted through the right ventricular cavity and causes the pulmonary valve to open in presystole thus lessening the impact of the onset of ejection on the blood in the root of the pulmonary artery so that the ejection click disappears (Fig. 11b). The earlier during inspiration this occurs the more severe the stenosis (p. 110) and this feature therefore provides a means of estimating by auscultation the severity of the pulmonary valve stenosis. *Aortic ejection clicks* also occur in the absence of any aortic valve abnormality in hypertension, dilatation of the aortic root and in normal middle-aged and elderly people. The genesis of the ejection click in this situation is less clearly established but as the ejection click occurs at the moment the aortic valve opens fully and ejection into the aorta commences it is probable that the sound is the result of vibrations set up in the root of the aorta, possibly in association with increased rigidity of the aortic wall.

A loud aortic systolic ejection click is heard in *pulmonary atresia* and in *coarctation of the aorta*. In coarctation the ejection click is probably due to the presence of a bicuspid aortic valve which also occurs frequently in this condition.

An aortic ejection click is usually best heard at the left sternal border and often at the apex whereas a pulmonary ejection click is usually loudest in the second left intercostal space but is also often quite well heard at the left sternal border.

Mid or late systolic clicks

Not uncommonly a systolic click is audible in mid or late

systole. Its timing is such that it is unlikely to be confused with an ejection click or with splitting of the first sound but as it produces a triple rhythm it may be confused with a true gallop rhythm and may cause difficulty in distinguishing systole from diastole, with resultant misinterpretation of the other heart sounds and any murmurs present.

Exocardial (*pericardial*) clicks arise outside of the heart and are probably due to pericardial scarring. They may occur anywhere in the praecordium and sometimes replace a previous pericardial rub during the healing phase of pericarditis. They can however occur without any evidence or history of heart disease.

Since the ready availability of echocardiography, *mitral valve prolapse* has been identified as a not uncommon cause of a mid-systolic click. It is usually best heard at or near the apex and may be followed by an apical late systolic murmur. On echocardiography the click can be seen to coincide with the beginning of the prolapse of the valve (Fig. 12). Its mechanism is not fully understood but is probably associated with vibrations set up in the mitral valve leaflet as it balloons back into the left atrium. Although this is usually a benign condition sometimes quite severe mitral regurgitation can accompany the prolapse.

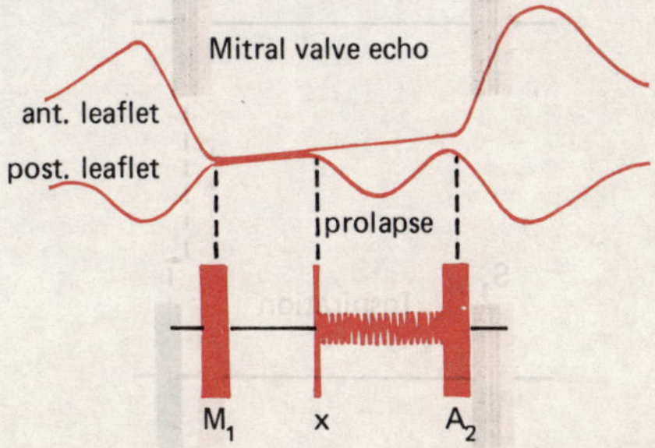

Fig. 12 The mid-systolic click (X) and late systolic murmur of mitral valve prolapse.

The mild cases of prolapse with or without a late systolic murmur are often accompanied by palpitation and non-anginal cardiac pain.

SPLITTING OF THE SECOND HEART SOUND

In routine examination of the heart particular attention should be paid to the second heart sound at the base. In difficult cases, when the diagnosis is not immediately obvious, very useful information may be obtained by attention to detail.

Physiological splitting

The normal second sound (S_2) has two components, as explained on p. 45, which can be referred to as A_2 and P_2 respectively, and every effort should be made to distinguish them by listening throughout the respiratory cycle. Usually the two components separate during inspiration and fuse on expiration so that if splitting can be heard on expiration it is almost always abnormal.

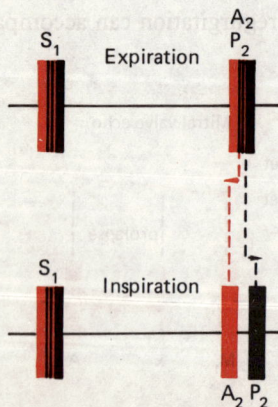

Fig. 13 Normal splitting of the second sound with respiration.

During inspiration the normally negative intrathoracic pressure becomes still more negative with resultant increase in venous return from the extrathoracic vessels to the right cardiac chambers. During deep inspiration this is exaggerated, stroke volume is increased, right ventricular systole is prolonged and pulmonary valve closure further delayed.

This is in contrast to the absence of any differential effect on *intra*thoracic structures which are equally affected by changes in pressure, so that the return of blood from the lungs to the left atrium is not similarly increased. In fact, expansion of the lungs results in a decrease in venous return to the *left* side of the heart and consequently left ventricular systole is shortened and aortic valve closure occurs slightly early. This combined movement of the two components of the second sound on inspiration results in their separation, often to a distance of about 0.04 s (Fig. 13).

While it is sometimes easier to ask the patient to take a long slow breath and then hold it *without straining*, then breathe out and hold it similarly in expiration, there is always a danger that the patient will unconsciously close his glottis and perform a Valsalva manoeuvre. This will produce marked changes in intrathoracic pressure which may then confuse the interpretation of the splitting of the second sound.

If separation of the two components is less than 0.03 s they cannot be distinguished and the sound will appear single.

Pathological splitting

'Normal' splitting — A_2P_2

Abnormally wide splitting of the second heart sound is most often due to *delay in pulmonary valve closure* but sometimes results from *premature closure of the aortic valve*.

Delay in pulmonary valve closure may result from delayed activation of the RV or from prolongation of RV systole.

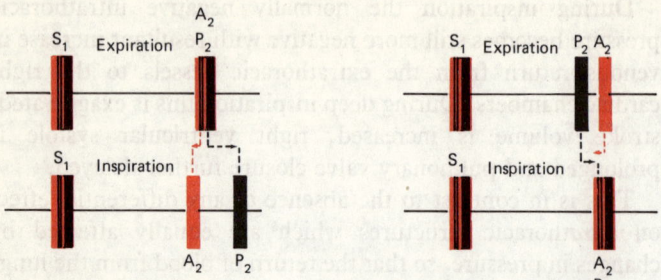

a. Pathological 'Normal' splitting
(Prolonged RV ejection)

b. Pathological Reversed splitting
(Prolonged LV ejection)

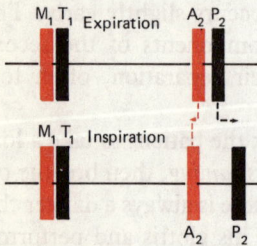

c. Right Bundle Branch Block
(Delayed RV ejection)

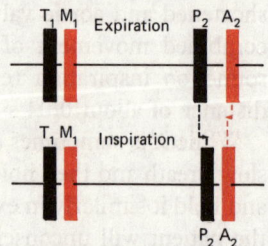

d. Left Bundle Branch Block
(Delayed LV ejection)

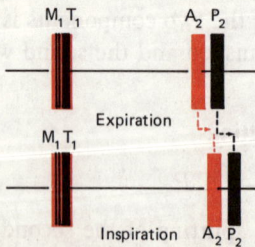

e. Fixed splitting
(Prolonged LV and RV ejection)

Fig. 14 Pathological splitting of the second heart sound.

Activation of the RV is delayed in right bundle branch block, resulting in a widely split second sound even in expiration. On inspiration the normal physiological prolongation of RV ejection further increases the degree of splitting (Fig. 14c).

Prolongation of RV systole may result from a relative increase in stroke volume compared with the LV as in a left-to-right shunt through an atrial septal defect or in pulmonary regurgitation, from obstruction to RV outflow or from impairment of RV function (Fig. 14a). In some such cases the degree of splitting cannot be further increased by deep inspiration and is described as being 'fixed'.

In summary, delay in pulmonary valve closure may result from delayed activation from right bundle branch block, from increased RV stroke volume, from obstruction to RV outflow or from RV failure.

Difficulty inevitably arises if one or other component of a split second sound is too faint to be heard with certainty or if it is obscured by a loud murmur.

Early aortic valve closure may result from decreased LV outflow into the aorta due to incompetence of the mitral valve or to a ventricular septal defect, when there is a 'double outlet' for the left ventricle.

Reversed (paradoxical) splitting — P_2A_2

Prolongation of LV ejection or delay in its activation may cause A_2 to fall later than P_2, giving rise to audible splitting of the second sound on expiration. During inspiration P_2 moves in the usual way but *towards* A_2 instead of away from it, resulting in a single sound. This is the reverse of normal and hence the term reversed or paradoxical splitting (Fig. 14b). The most frequent causes are obstruction to LV outflow at valvar or subvalvar level, impaired myocardial function as from infarction, severe aortic regurgitation with an increased stroke volume and left bundle branch block (Fig. 14d).

Fixed splitting of second sound

The term *fixed splitting* of S_2 is used when the two components remain separated by the same interval during inspiration and expiration. The classical example is in atrial septal defect. In this condition pulmonary valve closure is delayed due to the increased RV stroke volume which results from the left to right shunt giving rise to wide separation but, since the two atria are in free communication, they behave as one chamber, and the effect of inspiration is similar on the two sides of the heart (Fig. 14e).

CAUSES OF PATHOLOGICAL SPLITTING

'Normal' splitting — A_2P_2

Prolonged right ventricular ejection

Increased volume
    Anomalous pulmonary venous drainage
    Atrial septal defect (fixed splitting)
    Pulmonary regurgitation
Obstruction to outflow
    Pulmonary stenosis
Impaired contraction
    Congestive cardiomyopathy
    Cor pulmonale
    Massive pulmonary embolism
    RV myocardial infarction/ischaemia

Delayed right ventricular ejection

    Right bundle branch block
    Left ventricular ectopic beats

Reversed (paradoxical) splitting — P_2A_2

Prolonged left ventricular ejection

Increased volume
  Aortic regurgitation
  Patent ductus arteriosus
Obstruction to outflow
  Aortic stenosis
  Hypertrophic obstructive cardiomyopathy
Impaired contraction
  Ischaemic heart disease
  Hypertensive heart disease
  Congestive cardiomyopathy

Delayed left ventricular ejection

  Left bundle branch block
  Right ventricular ectopic beats
  Right ventricular pacing

Emphasis on the fixed nature of the splitting has led to under-emphasis of the fact that audible *expiratory splitting* is the abnormality which is most readily detected. Once the interval of splitting on expiration has been noted attention should then be paid to whether this interval changes on inspiration.

Fixed splitting may also be found in severe right heart failure, including the acute right heart failure which occurs with massive pulmonary embolism. In this situation, the right ventricle is already maximally loaded even on expiration and thus cannot significantly increase its filling on inspiration. The volume of blood to be ejected thus remains the same and the pulmonary component is delayed by a constant amount. For the same reason fixed splitting is heard occasionally in congestive cardiomyopathy, though in this condition normal and reversed splitting may also both occur depending on whether the right or the left ventricle is predominantly affected.

In right bundle branch block it is usually possible to detect some increase in splitting on inspiration but this is not always the case, especially if there is right heart failure.

Single second sound

The second heart sound will appear single if the two components are separated by less than 0.03 s. This is not uncommon especially with increasing age.

In moderate aortic stenosis prolongation of LV ejection may result in superimposition of A_2 on P_2, producing a single second sound. In more severe stenosis the greater prolongation of ejection may result in reversed splitting (p. 79). In severe calcific aortic stenosis, A_2 is frequently inaudible and the second sound consisting only of P_2 is single and soft.

Likewise in severe pulmonary stenosis P_2 in addition to being delayed may become inaudible although it can usually be recorded on the phonocardiogram. In this case a single second sound consisting of A_2 is heard but is as a rule louder than the single sound in severe aortic stenosis.

When a ventricular septal defect is very large as in the rare congenital condition, Eisenmenger's Complex, or when the interventricular septum is absent as in univentricular heart, the two ventricles behave physiologically as a single chamber, aortic and pulmonary closure occur simultaneously and S_2 is thus single and loud.

In the congenital malformation known as a common truncus arteriosus there is only one functioning valve and hence a single sound.

Differential diagnosis of split second sound

Splitting of the second heart sound in expiration must be differentiated from an opening snap, gallop rhythm with a third heart sound, a pericardial 'knock' or, occasionally, a late systolic click.

An opening snap from mitral stenosis may be loud in the pulmonary area and sometimes over the whole precordium. With severe stenosis, differentiation from splitting may be difficult because the snap may occur as early as 0.06 s after A_2, which is within the normal range of splitting of S_2 in inspiration. Identification can be achieved if it is possible to distinguish both components of S_2 in addition to the snap. A snap is usually followed by a mitral diastolic murmur, but it may be necessary to listen *precisely* over the apex with the patient lying in the left lateral position. A mitral diastolic murmur may be present without a preceding snap if the valve is sclerotic or calcified or if there is dominant regurgitation. Sometimes only a snap is audible after valvotomy.

The interval between S_2 and a snap is usually between 0.06 and 0.10 s, and that between S_2 and a third sound between 0.12 and 0.16 s. A third heart sound can usually be distinguished from a delayed P_2 by its later occurrence, lower pitch and duller character. When associated with mitral regurgitation it may be immediately followed by a short decrescendo mitral diastolic murmur due to increased flow.

A pericardial 'knock' is usually sharp and the distance from the commencement of S_2 may be as short as 0.10 s. It may therefore simulate fixed splitting of S_2 or an opening snap.

Sometimes, of course, splitting of S_2 is present as well as one or other of these additional sounds. Differentiation is usually possible by taking all factors into consideration, including the findings on palpation.

GALLOP RHYTHM

'This particularly rapid, unintelligible patter
Isn't generally heard and if it is it doesn't matter.'
— W. S. Gilbert.

So sang Gilbert a hundred years ago, and so might some sing today about gallop rhythm, particularly perhaps physicians brought up before the days of modern analysis but not, let us hope, the student who has the opportunity to start aright.

Classification

Third heart sound	Left ventricular
	Right ventricular
	Physiological
	Pathological
	Pericardial Knock
Fourth heart sound	Left atrial
	Right atrial
Summation gallop	
Quadruple gallop	

Much of the confusion stems from the different meanings intended by different authors when using the terms *triple rhythm* and *gallop rhythm*. Triple rhythm signifies that three heart sounds can be heard instead of the usual two. Used in this literal sense the term is so all-embracing as to be of no practical value. Furthermore there are occasions when all four heart sounds can be heard (the so-called quadruple gallop).

The term gallop rhythm is used when, in addition to the two main heart sounds there is present a third and/or a fourth heart sound. All other added sounds such as opening snaps and midsystolic clicks should be referred to by name and not included under the term gallop rhythm.

All added sounds of true gallop rhythm thus fall during diastole.

The terms third and fourth heart sound are, by convention, used respectively for the additional sound in early diastole associated with rapid ventricular filling and that occurring in late diastole (presystole) and dependent upon atrial systole.

Confusion over terminology from differences of opinion can easily be avoided by invariably qualifying the term 'gallop rhythm' by its cause, such as gallop rhythm from the addition of a physiological or pathological third heart sound.

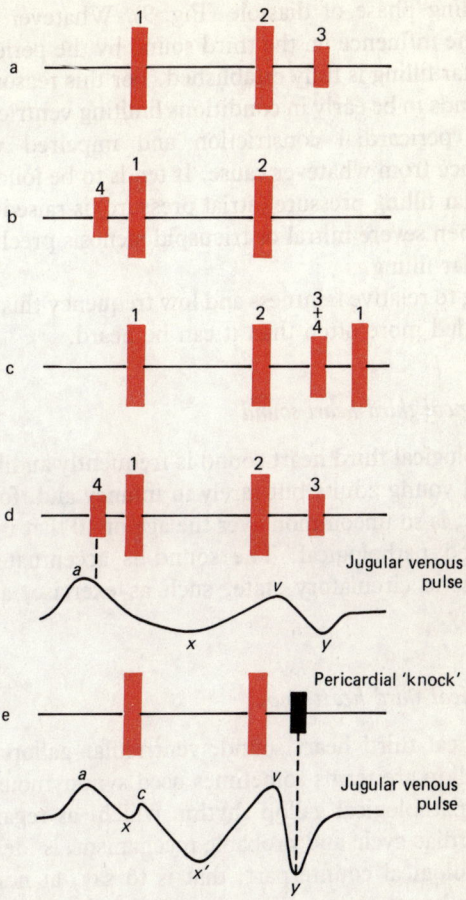

Fig. 15 Gallop rhythm. a. Early diastolic gallop due to a third sound.
b. Presystolic gallop due to a fourth sound. c. Summation gallop due to
superimposition of third and fourth sounds. d. Quadruple gallop due to the
presence of both third and fourth sounds heard separately. e. Pericardial
'knock'.

is beginning its partial closure movement at the end of the rapid filling phase of diastole (Fig. 9). Whatever the mechanism, the influence on the third sound by the period of rapid ventricular filling is fully established. For this reason the third sound tends to be early in conditions limiting ventricular filling such as pericardial constriction and impaired ventricular compliance from whatever cause. It tends to be loud when the ventricular filling pressure (atrial pressure) is raised and is not heard when severe mitral or tricuspid stenosis precludes rapid ventricular filling.

Owing to relative faintness and low frequency this sound can be recorded more often than it can be heard.

Physiological third heart sound

A physiological third heart sound is frequently audible in children and young adults but rarely in infancy and, for practical purposes, is so uncommon over the age of 40 that it should be considered pathological. The sound is accentuated by any hyperkinetic circulatory state, such as exercise, anaemia or pregnancy.

Pathological third heart sound

Pathological third heart sound, ventricular gallop and rapid filling gallop are terms sometimes used synonymously for one form of pathological gallop rhythm which, as regards timing in the cardiac cycle and probable mechanism, is identical with its physiological counterpart, that is to say, at normal heart rates it is heard early in diastole and shortly after the second sound. It may be loudest at the apex or near the sternum, depending on which ventricle is involved, and also on other factors such as cardiac enlargement, rotation or displacement. A *left sided* third sound may result from systemic hypertension, myocardial infarction or any form of cardiomyopathy causing left ventricular failure. It is commonly heard in severe mitral regurgitation and in ventricular septal defects.

A *right sided* third sound occurs frequently in massive pulmonary embolism and certain forms of cardiomyopathy, but rarely from tricuspid regurgitation.

The sound is of a dull, low frequency quality and may be accompanied by a palpable impulse. It usually indicates *myocardial failure* from any cause.

Differential diagnosis is discussed on p. 95.

PRESYSTOLIC (ATRIAL) GALLOP RHYTHM

Fourth heart sound

An added sound in presystole, usually referred to as the fourth heart sound, can frequently be recorded as a phonocardiographic event of low intensity and low frequency. It appears just after the beginning of the P wave and before the R wave of the electro-cardiogram and coincides with the '*a*' wave of the jugular venous pulse (Fig. 15). Like the third sound, the fourth heart sound is dependent on filling of the ventricle but whereas the third sound is associated with passive early rapid filling of the ventricle in diastole the fourth sound depends on active presystolic filling of the ventricle brought about by atrial systole. Consequently it is lost with the development of atrial fibrillation whereas the third sound is unaffected by this. The fourth sound can be seen on echophonocardiography to occur after atrial systole has fully opened the A–V valve and the valve is beginning to close again (see Fig. 9).

As with the third sound there is now a large amount of evidence to suggest that the fourth sound is due to vibrations set up in the respective A–V valve apparatus (valve leaflets, chordae and papillary muscles) when the ventricle resists further distension. The fourth sound is thus an indicator of alteration of ventricular compliance and will be loud when decreased compliance brings about a more abrupt limitation to ventricular filling. If as in very severe aortic regurgitation the mitral valve fails to open with atrial systole no fourth sound is recorded.

Physiological fourth heart sound

The low-pitched vibrations which form the atrial component of the first heart sound cannot *usually* be distinguished in health. In a few normal persons, and especially when there is delay in A–V conduction (as reflected in prolongation of the P–R interval of the electrocardiogram), this sound may be audible immediately before the first heart sound. It differs in quality from splitting of the first sound (due to asynchronous closure of the mitral and tricuspid valves) in that the latter is composed of two similar high-pitched sounds. That atrial contraction can produce an audible sound is readily demonstrated in patients with complete heart block, when there is dissociation between atrial and ventricular contractions. In such cases independent, irregular atrial sounds can often be heard.

Pathological fourth heart sound

A distinct, presystolic gallop rhythm is frequently heard in patients with *left sided heart disease*, particularly in those with left ventricular hypertrophy from systemic hypertension, aortic stenosis or hypertrophic cardiomyopathy or with reduced left ventricular compliance from any cause such as congestive cardiomyopathy or myocardial infarction.

In *right sided heart disease* a presystolic gallop rhythm may occur from pulmonary hypertension, pulmonary embolism or reduced right ventricular compliance from any cause.

In many patients the clarity of this added sound and its distance from the first heart sound decreases with clinical improvement and in others, especially with systemic hypertension, there may be no change over many years without clinical deterioration. The sound, in fact, may be heard in patients with left ventricular hypertrophy from *symptomless* hypertension. Usually it reflects either left ventricular failure with a raised end diastolic pressure in the left ventricle or decreased compliance of the ventricular walls from hypertrophy. The sound may be *increased* by exercise or elevation of the legs, all of which enhance venous return to the heart, or *decreased* by the Valsalva manoeuvre, sitting upright or venous occlusion tourniquets applied to the thighs which restricts venous return. A right sided fourth sound is often increased by inspiration because of the greater venous return to the right atrium with the increased negative intrathoracic pressure on inspiration but in right heart failure the loading of the right ventricle may be maximal even on expiration, in which case the fourth sound will be unaffected by inspiration. The left sided fourth sound will either be unaffected by respiration or maximal on expiration due to the diminished venous return to the left atrium during inspiration.

A pathological fourth sound is often inconstant and may, for example, appear during an attack of angina and disappear after its relief.

At other times, with worsening of the patient's condition and in particular with the onset of overt cardiac failure, a fourth sound may disappear to be replaced by a third sound, only to reappear with subsequent improvement and disappearance of the third sound.

Occasionally third and fourth sounds are both present, giving rise to a quadruple gallop (Fig. 15d).

SUMMATION GALLOP

Summation gallop signifies the superimposition of atrial and ventricular added sounds. With a heart rate of around 120 beats per minute, shortening of diastole results in the third sound of one heart cycle being superimposed on the fourth sound of the next cycle (Fig. 15c). The sound thus produced occurs approximately in mid diastole (it is actually usually slightly after mid diastole but this is difficult to recognise because of the tachycardia). Because it consists of two super-imposed sounds, it is louder than either the third or fourth sound would be if heard separately.

Because of this, a summation gallop is probably the variety of pathological gallop rhythm most easily recognised and its association with tachycardia from ventricular failure is respon-sible for the gloomy prognosis so often associated with gallop rhythm.

When the P–R interval of the electrocardiogram is prolonged, producing a greater interval between the fourth sound and the following first sound, summation will occur at a lower heart rate and in cases of marked increase in P–R interval may even occur at a normal heart rate.

Summation of the two added sounds can, of course, only be proved by their separation with slowing of the heart rate. This can sometimes be achieved by carotid sinus massage or may occur spontaneously with improvement in the cardiac failure.

GALLOP RHYTHM IN CONSTRICTIVE PERICARDITIS

A characteristic added sound early in diastole, somewhat similar in timing but louder, higher pitched and a little earlier (around 0.12 s) than other third heart sounds is often heard in advanced cases of constrictive pericarditis and may be accompanied by a palpable impulse. It is sometimes referred to as a pericardial 'knock' but it is doubtful whether this term, which implies that it is different from a third sound, is really justified. Its mechanism of production is probably the same as that of a third sound and both the sound and palpable impulse are probably due to a combination of the elevated atrial pressure and the abrupt limitation of filling produced by the unyielding qualities of the thickened and often calcified pericardium.

It is associated with a prominent *y* descent in the jugular venous pulse which is due to the initially high venous pressure at the time of opening of the tricuspid valve and an equally rapid rebound from the *y* trough to a *z* plateau produced by the limitation of ventricular filling (Fig. 15e).

Differential diagnosis is from other types of third heart sound and an opening snap (p. 95).

OPENING SNAP OF THE MITRAL VALVE

The opening snap of the mitral valve is a characteristic, high-pitched sound best heard with a diaphragm chest piece and usually loudest between the apex beat and the left sternal border. It may be audible over a wide area of the chest wall.

In timing it occurs early in diastole (0.05 to 0.12 s) after the beginning of the second heart sound and shortly after the peak of the V wave of the jugular venous pulse, that is to say, immediately after the opening of the A–V valves. Echophono-cardiography has demonstrated that the opening snap occurs when the A–V valve reaches its widest open position (see Fig. 9). The mechanism responsible for the opening snap is probably very similar to that responsible for the ejection click (p. 72) namely the piston-like effect of the opening of the valve setting up vibrations in the blood immediately down-stream from the valve which are transmitted to the valve apparatus and its surrounding structure. Whatever the actual cause of the snap, its coincidence with the opening of the A–V valve is beyond any doubt and factors which accelerate or delay the opening of the valve result in an earlier or later opening snap respectively. If left atrial pressure is high, as is often the case in severe mitral stenosis, the valve will open sooner than otherwise. Consequently the interval between the aortic component of the second sound and the opening snap (2-OS) has been recommended as a guide to severity. However, taken in isolation, this is unreliable because factors other than the degree of stenosis also affect left atrial pressure, including left atrial volume and compliance, the cardiac output (which is itself influenced by a number of factors) and the presence or absence of mitral regurgitation or of left ventricular failure. Nevertheless, when considered along with other evidence of mitral stenosis it provides a useful guide to the severity of the stenosis.

An opening snap can be heard in most patients with mitral stenosis of any degree whether or not this is complicated by regurgitation, provided that at least one leaflet is still mobile. With heavily calcified or sclerotic, and hence immobile, cusps, the snap may be absent, muffled or soft. An opening snap is usually immediately followed by a mitral diastolic murmur. However with very mild mitral stenosis and after a good mitral valvotomy, only a snap may be audible. When the mitral valve has been replaced by one of the mechanical prostheses such as the caged-ball type, the opening snap which occurs when the ball reaches the limit of its opening excursion at the end of the cage, is often very loud. Auscultation in such a patient provides the student with a very useful guide to the timing and character of an opening snap. With the tissue xenograft prostheses, the opening snap is much softer and may be completely absent. Provided the prosthesis is functioning normally and is of adequate size, there is no mitral diastolic murmur.

Stenosis of a mitral valve whose leaflets are still mobile and pliant is accompanied by a loud first sound and a clear opening snap but the converse is not always true. A clear opening snap may be produced by a valve with one mobile leaflet and the other rendered completely immobile by calcification. Furthermore even though the leaflets of the valve may be mobile there is no auscultatory sign by which one can detect subvalvar fusion of the chordae, a condition which is often present when restenosis has occurred after an initially successful mitral valvotomy. For this reason it is unwise to rely on auscultatory findings alone to decide whether the surgeon will be able to achieve a successful mitral valvotomy.

As the mitral opening snap may be heard over a wide area and is sometimes best heard at the left sternal border and as rheumatic tricuspid stenosis almost never occurs without coexisting mitral valve disease, it is very difficult to distinguish between a mitral and tricuspid opening snap. The tricuspid opening snap is usually earlier and often higher pitched than the mitral and may be louder on inspiration because of the increased venous return to the right atrium. When both mitral and tricuspid valves have been replaced by mechanical prostheses, it is often possible to distinguish both components of the first sound and both opening snaps occurring very close together.

Mitral and tricuspid opening snaps may occur in the absence of valve stenosis for example, in the case of the mitral valve, with hyperkinetic circulatory states such as thyrotoxicosis, with mitral regurgitation, right to left shunt at atrial level and A–V block and in the tricuspid valve with atrial septal defect. All of these conditions produce an increased volume and/or velocity of flow in early diastole across the respective A–V valve. However such instances are uncommon.

Differential diagnosis is chiefly from wide splitting of the second heart sound and an early third heart sound.

DIFFERENTIAL DIAGNOSIS OF THIRD HEART SOUND, PERICARDIAL KNOCK AND OPENING SNAP

A third heart sound, pericardial knock and opening snap each occurs as an extra sound early in diastole and may cause difficulty in differentiation unless all associated circumstances are taken into account. There is overlap in precise timing.

An opening snap from mitral stenosis usually occurs between 0.05 and 0.12 s after the second heart sound and is almost always followed by a mitral diastolic murmur. A diastolic murmur may not be audible if blood flow is greatly reduced by a high pulmonary vascular resistance, in which case there will be evidence of pulmonary hypertension (p. 153).

A pathological third sound usually occurs later than an opening snap (0.12 to 0.16 s) or pericardial knock, and is of a duller quality and may or may not be followed by a decrescendo diastolic murmur from increased blood flow. It is an important sign of severity in mitral regurgitation and may be associated with any form of myocardial failure, other signs of which should be sought.

A pericardial knock occurs slightly earlier in diastole than other third sounds but more closely resembles a snap in quality, and is not associated with a murmur.

In all three conditons atrial fibrillation may be present.

Splitting of the first and second heart sounds is not included in the term gallop rhythm because they are normal components of these sounds.

Where doubt is felt over classification, clarity can be ensured by qualifying the term gallop rhythm with an additional comment, for example gallop rhythm due to the addition of a third or fourth sound or a pericardial knock. A third sound refers to the one occurring early in diastole and the fourth sound to that occurring late in diastole (presystolic). All other added sounds such as ejection and midsystolic clicks and opening snaps, sometimes included under the broader term of 'triple rhythm' should not be included in 'gallop rhythm' but described by the name of the added sound.

4

Murmurs

*'Give me a calm and thankful heart,
From every murmur free.'*
— from a hymn by Anne Steele, 1760.

The difference between a sound and a murmur is that the former is due to sudden alteration in the speed of blood flow whereas a murmur results from turbulence or vortices in the blood stream (p. 51).

A murmur is of longer duration and usually of higher frequency than a sound. The principal factors which influence its quality are velocity of flow, density and viscosity of the blood, changes of calibre as regards blood flow through the heart, valves or large vessels, and irregularities of the endothelium.

It is remarkable that blood flow through the heart, round bends and past protuberances in valves should be so silent, and not surprising that minor irregularities of no structural consequence should sometimes cause eddies and be associated with a murmur. Murmurs may arise from a normal amount of blood flowing through a narrowed orifice, as from valvar stenosis, or from a larger than normal amount of blood flowing through a normal sized orifice, as in the so-called 'flow' murmurs.

Intracardiac phonocardiography has demonstrated that the murmur is conducted in the blood stream in the direction of the blood flow producing the murmur. However vibrations set up in the surrounding structures may produce clinical conduction of a murmur behind as well as beyond the obstruction.

A similar effect is produced by a relatively narrow vessel opening into a wider one, as in dilatation of the first part of the aorta or pulmonary artery.

Murmurs may be heard in systole or diastole or may be continuous throughout systole and diastole.

Diastolic murmurs are always due to organic disease and continuous murmurs usually so, but a systolic murmur is often present not only without functional disability but without any clinical, radiographic or electrocardiographic evidence of organic heart disease or obvious cause other than normal blood flow.

In all cases the area over which a murmur is heard should be noted and also the position of maximal intensity, the direction of apparent conduction, the intensity (graded), the quality (using simple adjectives) and, where possible, the precise timing in systole or diastole.

It should also be noted whether it is associated with a palpable thrill and if there is any abnormality of the heart sounds.

In cases of doubt, and when of clinical importance and not just a matter of curiosity, echocardiography, phonocardiography, radiography, electrocardiography and other accessory methods of examination may be required before a firm conclusion as to significance can be drawn.

Factors influencing the character and loudness of murmurs

The qualities of a murmur depend on its spectrum of frequencies.

A low pitched diastolic murmur is usually due to low velocity flow through the mitral and tricuspid valves, whereas a high-pitched blowing systolic murmur, such as that from mitral regurgitation or a ventricular septal defect, is due to a relatively narrow jet of blood passing at high velocity from a high pressure to a low pressure chamber.

The chief factor influencing loudness is the rate of flow through the orifice or vessel responsible for the murmur.

Loudness will also depend to some extent on the proximity of the source of origin to the chest wall and on intervening lung which varies with the phases of respiration.

Changes in flow can be brought about physiologically by respiration or posture and by hyperkinetic states such as hyperthroidism, anaemia and pregnancy. Conversely, cardiac failure, pulmonary hypertension and hypothyroidism are conditions which reduce blood flow.

Variation in flow can also be achieved by use of the Valsalva manoeuvre and by drugs which influence vascular resistance, such as amyl nitrite or phenylephrine.

SYSTOLIC MURMURS

Classification

Forward flow: Aortic
(Ejection)
             Aortic sclerosis
             Obstruction to left ventricular outflow
                Aortic valve stenosis
                Supravalvar aortic stenosis
                Subvalvar aortic stenosis
                Hypertrophic obstructive cardiomyopathy
             Increased flow
                Physiological
                Aortic regurgitation
             Pulmonary
                Obstruction to right ventricular outflow
                Pulmonary valve stenosis
                Pulmonary infundibular stenosis
             Increased flow

	Physiological
	Left to right shunts
Backward flow:	Mitral regurgitation
(*Regurgitant*)	Tricuspid regurgitation
	Ventricular septal defect
Miscellaneous:	Arterial stenosis
	Patent ductus (with pulmonary hypertension)
	Parasternal (idiopathic, 'innocent')

Systolic murmurs fall between the first and second heart sounds. They may occur in early, mid or late systole or occupy the whole of systole.

A systolic murmur may be due to various acquired or congenital defects or occur as an isolated finding unassociated with organic disease when they are sometimes termed innocent, incidental or functional (p. 120).

If a systolic murmur can be heard its characteristics should be noted, as described above, and also whether there is any accompanying thrill, diastolic murmur, change in heart sounds or other evidence of structural change.

A general classification of systolic murmurs is necessary and for this purpose they can be divided into two main groups: *ejection*, due to forward flow, that is in the normal direction, and *regurgitant*, due to backward flow in an abnormal direction. A systolic murmur cannot always be placed with certainty in one or other of these categories and in this case the auscultator should keep an open mind about the origin of the murmur and make due note of this when describing the murmur. However for a clear understanding of heart sounds and particularly of heart murmurs it is essential to relate what is heard to the underlying mechanics and physiology of the heart action. With this approach it is often possible to deduce what type of murmur can be expected from a given anatomical or physiological situation, thus avoiding a large amount of 'parrot fashion' learning and also of stupid errors such as ascribing an ejection type of systolic murmur, indicating forward flow, to an A–V valve.

To acquire this understanding it is best to relate the heart sounds and murmurs to the relevant pressure curves during the heart cycle. These changes and their associated auscultatory findings will now be reviewed in detail. For simplicity we will consider only the events taking place in the left side of the heart but it must be remembered that exactly the same principles apply to the right side of the heart.

EJECTION SYSTOLIC MURMURS

With the onset of ventricular systole, left ventricular pressure very soon rises above that in left atrium, the mitral valve closes and the mitral component of the first heart sound is produced (Fig. 16). At this stage the aortic valve has not yet opened and this will only take place when the left ventricular pressure rises above the level of pressure in the aorta. Once this happens the aortic valve opens and if present the ejection click is heard. This marks the onset of ejection of blood from the heart and the preceding interval between the first sound and the ejection click corresponds to the isovolumic contraction phase of the left ventricle. With the onset of ejection of blood from the left ventricle into the aorta through, for example, a stenosed aortic valve, an ejection murmur will be heard commencing with the ejection click if present but, in the absence of an ejection click, still separated from the first sound by the silent interval of isovolumic contraction. As the flow through the aortic valve increases to a maximum at the peak of ventricular systole, so the systolic murmur is crescendo in quality and reaches its maximum at that time. With subsequent relaxation of the left ventricle flow through the aortic valve diminishes again and the murmur becomes progressively softer. At the point at which the left ventricular pressure falls below that in aorta the dicrotic notch on the aortic pulse wave is inscribed and the

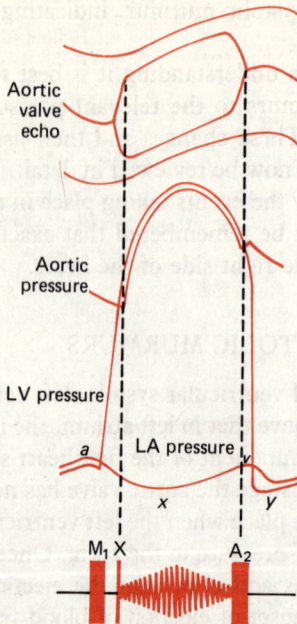

Fig. 16 Aortic systolic ejection murmur. The timing of the heart sounds, ejection click and murmur is shown in relation to the changes in left heart pressures and the opening and closing of the aortic valve as seen on the M-mode echocardiogram.

aortic component of the second sound is heard. With closure of the aortic valve no further ejection is possible and therefore the aortic ejection murmur must end with the second sound. However, with severe obstruction to LV outflow and delay in aortic valve closure, there may be reversed splitting of the second sound (p. 79), and the aortic murmur may be heard beyond the pulmonary component. For similar reasons the murmur of pulmonary valve stenosis may extend beyond the aortic component to end with the pulmonary component of the second sound which may be delayed by prolongation of RV systole.

Regurgitant systolic murmurs

With the onset of ventricular systole the pressure in the left ventricle rises above that in the left atrium producing, as described earlier, the first heart sound (Fig. 17). Immediately the pressure in the left ventricle is greater than that in the left atrium a driving force exists capable of causing flow of blood through an incompetent mitral valve. The usual regurgitant murmur therefore begins immediately with the first sound and may to some extent swamp it. As the pressure in the left ventricle rapidly becomes much greater than that in the left atrium, and remains so throughout systole, the regurgitant

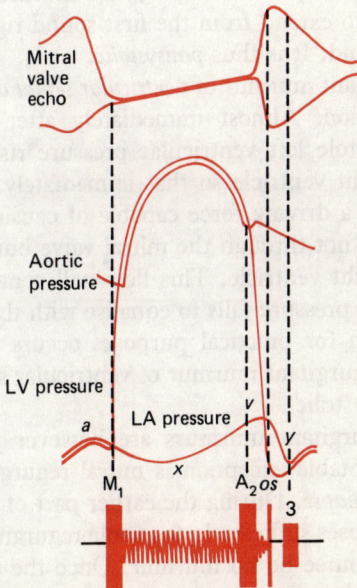

Fig. 17 Mitral pansystolic (regurgitant) murmur. The timing of the heart sounds, opening snap and the pansystolic murmur is shown in relation to the changes in left heart pressures and the closure and opening of the mitral valve as seen on the M-mode echocardiogram.

flow remains much more constant than in the case of forward flow. Consequently, the regurgitant murmur remains of approximately the same intensity throughout systole. The murmur will continue until the left ventricular pressure falls again to equalise with the left atrial pressure at which time the driving force causing the regurgitant flow will cease and at the same time the mitral valve will open again.

In theory the regurgitant murmur will then continue beyond the second sound to the point of opening of the mitral valve which may be signalled by an audible opening snap (Fig. 17). In practice it is usually difficult to detect the spilling over of the murmur through the second sound especially if there is no mitral opening snap. The regurgitant murmur is therefore usually heard to extend from the first sound right through to the second sound. It is thus *pansystolic*.

The regurgitant murmur of *ventricular septal defect* begins in a similar fashion. Almost immediately after the onset of ventricular systole left ventricular pressure rises faster than that in the right ventricle so that immediately after the first sound there is a driving force capable of causing regurgitant flow, this time not through the mitral valve but from the left ventricle to right ventricle. This flow will continue until the left ventricular pressure falls to equalise with that of the right ventricle which for practical purposes occurs at the second sound. The regurgitant murmur of ventricular septal defect is thus also pansystolic.

Not all regurgitant murmurs are however pansystolic in timing. The notable exception is mitral regurgitation due to *mitral valve prolapse*. During the earlier part of systole before the valve prolapses sufficiently to enable regurgitation to occur there will of course be no murmur. Once the conditions for regurgitation take effect the murmur will commence and will continue as with the pansystolic murmur through to the second sound or for however long the mitral valve prolapse permits regurgitation to occur.

At the bedside there are sometimes difficulties in identifying the true character of a murmur. It is sometimes not possible to hear both the heart sounds and the murmur in the one place. However usually careful auscultation from a number of different areas and the adoption of the technique of 'inching' the stethoscope from one area to another will usually enable all of the necessary features for classification of the murmur to be identified. The ejection murmur may not necessarily begin immediately after the onset of ejection of blood from the ventricle if the velocity of flow is initially insufficient to produce a murmur. Some ejection murmurs thus occupy only the mid portion of systole but usually they continue with diminishing intensity up to the aortic component of the second sound. A notable exception to the latter is however the murmur of *hypertrophic obstructive cardiomyopathy* where the ejection murmur is characteristically short and may end well before the second sound. With an inaudible aortic component of the second sound due to calcification the exact point of termination of the murmur may be difficult to determine.

These facts need not confuse the beginner and are mentioned to stimulate interest and to illustrate principles. In practice, when surgical treatment is under consideration the precise nature and severity of a structural defect must be determined by considering all available information. Sometimes this must include special laboratory investigations. Often, however, accurate interpretation by physical signs will suffice.

BASAL SYSTOLIC MURMURS

Basal systolic murmurs most often derive from the aortic or pulmonary valve. Sometimes they are transmitted from elsewhere, for example, mitral regurgitation with a jet directed upwards and medially rather than backwards.

Aortic systolic murmurs

The most frequent cause for a systolic murmur, which is loudest in the true aortic area (p. 48), is obstruction to left ventricular outflow at the valve. Less commonly obstruction is below, and rarely, above the valve.

A similar murmur may be due to valve sclerosis without stenosis, to relative stenosis from dilatation of the ascending aorta or to increased left ventricular stroke volume.

Aortic valve stenosis

Characteristically the murmur of aortic valve stenosis is harsh and loudest in midsystole because this corresponds to the period of maximal blood flow. On the phonocardiogram the configuration is often that of a diamond (Fig. 16). An aortic systolic murmur may be loudest to the right of the upper sternal border, over the sternum, down the left sternal border or sometimes even at the apex. Often, but by no means always, it is audible over the carotid arteries. Even when the murmur is not loudest to the right of the upper sternum, its origin may be recognised because it is also audible in this region and has similar timing.

The *quality* of the murmur is often more musical towards the apex, a dissociation which was first noticed by Gallavardin.

If the cusps are sclerotic or calcified, A_2 may be faint or absent. If only P_2 can be heard, it may be possible to appreciate by ear that the murmur ends before it. Usually it can be appreciated that there is a distinct gap between the first heart sound and the beginning of the murmur. However, in some cases one or other or both heart sounds cannot be heard, making precise timing impossible except by phonocardiography when simultaneous recordings can be recorded from several areas. Also the position in systole of maximal intensity depends on the degree of obstruction, being later with severe stenosis.

It is important to emphasise that the loudness of the murmur bears no close relationship to the degree of obstruction. In fact intensity is usually greatest with moderate stenosis. In severe cases, especially if there is left ventricular failure, the murmur may be faint or disappear.

There may or may not be an accompanying thrill but the intensity of the murmur does not always correspond to that of the thrill. Occasionally, even with a harsh murmur and thrill, there is no pressure gradient across the valve.

If the cusps are rigid and immobile there is usually an early diastolic murmur from associated aortic regurgitation.

The causes of aortic valve stenosis are rheumatic fever, a congenital dome-shaped deformity or a congenital bicuspid valve with sclerosis or calcification.

Obstruction to left ventricular outflow is sometimes at sub-valvar level. This may be due to muscular hypertrophy of the septum (*hypertrophic obstructive cardiomyopathy*) or occasionally to a congenital fibrous diaphragm or musculofibrous ring.

Supravalvar stenosis may also occur as a congenital malformation of the ascending aorta.

These conditions should be suspected if there are atypical features for valve stenosis, such as the absence of an ejection click in the absence of calcification or if the murmur and thrill are lower or higher in position than is usual for valvar stenosis.

Sclerosis of the cusps without significant stenosis is a common cause for an aortic systolic murmur in the elderly, especially in males.

A similar murmur may be found in apparently healthy young persons from a congenitally malformed and usually bicuspid valve. In a proportion (unknown) of such cases, progressive sclerosis or calification is responsible for severe valvar stenosis in later life.

Increased blood flow from a large stroke output, as in aortic regurgitation, may also be responsible for a systolic murmur and be present without any gradient across the valve.

Dilatation of the first part of the aorta with consequent relative stenosis of the valve may likewise result in sufficient turbulence to produce a murmur.

If the classical clinical features are present, a systolic murmur, maximal in the *conventional* aortic area, is most often due to aortic valve stenosis but, as discussed above, there are other causes for such a murmur. Also an aortic systolic murmur may be audible anywhere over the *true* aortic area or at the apex.

An associated aortic diastolic murmur favours valvar stenosis but may also occur with subvalvar stenosis due to a congenital diaphragm. An ejection click provides strong evidence that the stenosis is at valve level. If no ejection click is present, radioscopy of the valve for calcification should be carried out. If calcification is present the valvar origin of the murmur can be assumed but, if not present, then other possible causes such as subvalvar or supravalvar aortic stenosis should be carefully considered.

Dilatation of the ascending aorta also favours valvar stenosis.

It bears repetition that an aortic systolic murmur is *not* always loudest in the conventional aortic area or conducted into the carotids, its intensity bears *no* close relation to the severity of the underlying structural defect and it is *not* always accompanied by a thrill.

If there is no clinical, radiographic or electrocardiographic evidence of left ventricular enlargement or hypertrophy and the brachial pulse feels normal, the murmur is unlikely to be of sufficient haemodynamic significance to warrant further investigation or restriction of activities, but an annual review would be advisable.

In *coarctation of the aorta* the systolic murmur due to turbulence at the site of obstruction is usually loudest at the back over the spine and is often accompanied by murmurs over dilated collateral vessels. All of these murmurs are of the 'continuous' type (p. 143) but, if short, may be confused with a systolic ejection murmur. Furthermore a congenitally biscuspid aortic valve often accompanies coarctation of the aorta and this produces an aortic systolic ejection click and murmur anteriorly.

PULMONARY SYSTOLIC MURMURS

A pulmonary systolic murmur may be due to high flow across a normal valve, to valvar stenosis, to subvalvar obstruction to RV outflow, to supravalvar stenosis or merely to dilatation of the main pulmonary artery.

A pulmonary systolic murmur is probably the most frequent of all so-called functional or innocent murmurs.

Pulmonary valve stenosis

As with aortic stenosis, the characteristic murmur of pulmonary valve stenosis is usually loudest in midsystole, corresponding with the period of maximal ejection but there is no close relationship between the intensity of the murmur and the degree of obstruction. Like other systolic ejection murmurs that of pulmonary stenosis begins with the onset of ejection which may be marked by an ejection click (see Fig. 11). Whether or not a click is present there is the usual short silent period between the first sound and the onset of the murmur which corresponds to the isovolumic contraction phase of the ventricle. The peak of the murmur in systole depends on the degree of stenosis and whether or not there is an associated ventricular septal defect providing a double exit for blood from the right ventricle. In general the greater the degree of stenosis, the later the peak and the longer the duration of the murmur. There is often a systolic thrill. As with other murmurs of right heart origin, in the absence of cardiac failure the systolic murmur of pulmonary stenosis is louder on inspiration (p. 46).

As with aortic stenosis the presence of a systolic ejection click suggests strongly that the stenosis is at valve level. Whereas the ejection click of aortic valve stenosis is unaffected by respiration that of pulmonary stenosis may become softer or disappear on inspiration. Provided there is no associated atrial or ventricular septal defect the behaviour of the pulmonary ejection click provides a means of estimating the severity of the stenosis.

In mild pulmonary valve stenosis the filling resistance of the right ventricle is low and the *a* wave generated by atrial systole and transmitted into the right ventricle is of lower pressure than the pulmonary diastolic pressure and remains so even with the greater inflow of blood to the right atrium during inspiration. The pulmonary valve remains closed in presystole and is flung open early in right ventricular systole by the piston-like action of the blood at the commencement of ejection, producing the ejection click (see Fig. 11a). In moderate to severe pulmonary valve stenosis, the right atrial *a* wave is of higher pressure because of the greater filling resistance of the right ventricle but on expiration is still lower than the pulmonary artery diastolic pressure so that the pulmonary valve is still closed at the onset of ventricular systole and with ejection, click is again produced. With inspiration, the right atrial *a* wave pressure increases above the level of the pulmonary diastolic pressure. This *a* wave, transmitted through the right ventricle in presystole partially opens the pulmonary valve so that with the onset of ejection, the opening excursion of the valve and the piston-like thrust of the blood into the pulmonary artery is less forceful and insufficient to produce an ejection click. In this case, the click is heard on expiration but disappears at some point during inspiration (see Fig. 11b). In very severe pulmonary valve stenosis with marked right ventricular hypertrophy, the right atrial *a* wave is higher than the pulmonary diastolic pressure, even in expiration and when transmitted through the right ventricle opens the pulmonary valve in presystole throughout the respiratory cycle. There is thus no ejection click at any phase of respiration. In general therefore the tighter the stenosis the earlier will be ejection click disappear during inspiration.

As calcification of the pulmonary valve rarely occurs, absence of an ejection click at any phase of respiration should suggest the possibility of the stenosis being at other than valve level.

In severe pulmonary valve stenosis the second heart sound may be widely split, but the pulmonary component is usually faint or absent, depending on the degree of obstruction, so that the sound may appear single on auscultation.

Pulmonary valve stenosis is usually due to congenital fusion of the cusps.

Pulmonary infundibular stenosis

Subvalvar obstruction to right ventricular outflow occurs most commonly as part of the congenital abnormality known as Fallot's tetralogy in which pulmonary stenosis is associated with a large ventricular septal defect and over-riding of the aorta. It is relatively uncommon as an isolated abnormality in the absence of a ventricular septal defect. The stenosis is produced by a fibromuscular ring in the outflow tract of the right ventricle, below the pulmonary valve. The murmur and behaviour of the second sound may be identical with pulmonary valve stenosis but there is no systolic ejection click. The murmur of infundibular stenosis may be loudest in the third rather than the second left intercostal space.

Muscular obstruction of the right ventricular outflow tract may occur in systole as a result of marked right ventricular hypertrophy secondary to pulmonary valve stenosis or as part of a hypertrophic cardiomyopathy. Unlike the 'fixed' infundibular stenosis described above the purely muscular hypertrophy of the infundibulum produces systolic 'shut-down' of the right ventricular outflow tract with relaxation of the obstruction during diastole.

Supravalvar pulmonary stenosis

In this rare condition the obstruction occurs not at valve level but in the main pulmonary artery a short distance distal to the valve. The physical signs may be the same as with pulmonary valve stenosis except that an ejection click is usually absent unless there is associated pulmonary valve stenosis.

Occasionally an inspiratory systolic murmur in the pulmonary area is due to *pulmonary artery branch stenosis* which may affect either or both pulmonary arteries. The murmur of this condition is however of the 'continuous' type (p. 143).

Increased pulmonary blood flow

A systolic murmur from increased pulmonary blood flow across a normal valve may be associated with any hyperkinetic state, such as exercise, emotion, pregnancy, anemia or thyrotoxicosis. It is often heard in healthy young persons.

In congenital defects increased blood flow may be due to a left to right shunt from an atrial or ventricular septal defect.

A pulmonary systolic murmur is the most frequent murmur to be heard in the absence of valve disease and the most usual cause of what used to be called a *haemic murmur* (p. 122).

In atrial septal defect the intensity of the murmur depends not only on blood flow but on dilatation of the pulmonary artery, its proximity to the chest wall and on the degree of any associated pulmonary stenosis or pulmonary hypertension. An atrial septal defect may be suspected as the cause of the murmur if the second heart sound is clearly split during expiration and 'fixed' during inspiration (p. 80). There may also be an inspiratory diastolic murmur from increased flow across the tricuspid valve.

When due to increased flow across a normal valve the murmur tends to be more high pitched and blowing than in pulmonary stenosis. Like other right sided events it is often increased in intensity by inspiration.

Dilatation of pulmonary artery

Dilatation of the main pulmonary artery may occur as an isolated anomaly unassociated with heart disease and in such cases there is often a systolic murmur.

APICAL SYSTOLIC MURMURS

An apical systolic murmur is most often due to mitral regurgitation, of which there are a number of different causes, but may be transmitted and derive from aortic valve stenosis, subaortic obstruction to left ventricular outflow, tricuspid regurgitation, or a ventricular septal defect.

MITRAL REGURGITATION

Causes

Disease of valve cusps
Dilatation of the annulus or left ventricular chamber
Dysfunction or rupture of papillary muscle
Chordal rupture
Prolapse of valve cusps

Aetiology

Rheumatic fever
Left ventricular failure
Myocardial ischaemia or infarction
Infective endocarditis
Cardiomyopathy

Congenital malformation
Trauma
Left atrial myxoma

The characteristic murmur of mitral regurgitation is pansystolic, loudest at the apex and often well heard towards the left
axilla and lung base. The murmur is usually blowing or harsh
in character and may be accompanied by a systolic thrill.

As with other forms of valve disease, intensity of the
murmur is an unreliable guide to the severity of the defect but
severe regurgitation is likely to be present if there is also a third
heart sound (p. 86) which is often followed by a short,
decrescendo diastolic flow murmur (p. 141).

Less frequently the murmur occurs in late, mid or even early
systole.

The causes and aetiology of mitral regurgitation are listed
in the table.

Rheumatic mitral disease

This is probably still the most frequent cause even in the
Western world and usually the diagnosis is obvious. In the
absence of other evidence of heart disease, the finding on
routine examination of an apical systolic murmur always raises
the possibility of rheumatic mitral disease and this is a frequent
source of uncertainty in diagnosis. If there is a past history of
rheumatic fever or radiographic evidence of enlargement of the
left atrial appendage as well as the atrium itself, this diagnosis
must be made.

However, even if there is no other abnormality, it still
cannot be denied that minimal rheumatic heart disease is
present and, if possible, examination should be repeated at
intervals until it is certain that the situation is stationary.

Usually it is more important to avoid the error of diagnosing
organic heart disease when none is present than to ignore a

minor organic murmur, and this slight risk may reasonably be taken. In the occasional instance, infective endocarditis may subsequently develop in mild rheumatic mitral disease, but on balance there can be no question that this risk also should be accepted. From the practical point of view minor rheumatic mitral regurgitation in the absence of cardiac enlargement is of little haemodynamic significance and the patient should be reassured that the heart is healthy.

Regurgitant jet in mitral stenosis

In patients with mitral stenosis, especially with a sclerotic or calcified valve, it may not be possible for the cusps to come into perfect apposition in ventricular systole with a resultant regurgitant jet. This is often of no haemodynamic importance in comparison with the degree of obstruction. Such a murmur may be loud and is often high pitched or musical but usually not well conducted towards the left axilla. In such cases other physical signs denote dominant stenosis.

In other cases the relative degrees of mitral stenosis and regurgitation may be balanced or nearly so. Which lesion is dominant can often be decided by taking in account the findings on palpation and auscultation together with radiography, echocardiography and electrocardiography, but sometimes cardiac catheterisation with left ventricular angiography is necessary.

Apart from the haemodynamic aspects the significance of mitral regurgitation is often largely dependent upon its aetiology.

Functional mitral regurgitation

Functional mitral regurgitation, in the correct sense of the term, that is with normal valve cusps, may result from dilatation of the valve ring or from dilatation of the left ventricular chamber with 'pulling' on the chordae and papillary muscles.

Papillary muscle dysfunction or rupture

Dysfunction of the papillary muscles commonly results from coronary heart disease. This may occur acutely or be responsible for the finding of a mitral systolic murmur in the elderly.

Rupture of a papillary muscle may occur from acute myocardial infarction and require urgent surgical treatment. Differential diagnosis is from rupture of the interventricular septum and the distinction is important in relation to the timing of surgical treatment if this is indicated by the severity of symptoms.

Ruptured chordae tendineae

Rupture of chordae tendineae may occur spontaneously for no obvious reason or in patients with rheumatic heart disease or hypertension and the regurgitant jet may be in an unusual direction. With posterior rupture it may strike the left atrial wall opposite the root of the aorta giving rise to a systolic murmur and thrill in the right upper chest. This sometimes causes difficulty in differential diagnosis from an aortic murmur and the distinction is important because surgical treatment may be indicated. With anterior rupture the jet may be in the direction of the left sternal border and the murmur simulates a ventricular septal defect.

Mitral valve prolapse

With the availability of echocardiography it has been realised that mitral valve prolapse may occur in the absence of papillary muscle rupture or dysfunction, or of ruptured chordae tendineae. Often the degree of mitral regurgitation is mild and the murmur commences in mid-systole with or without a mid-systolic click (see Fig. 12). Such patients often present with a history of palpitation and vague chest pain not of anginal type. However occasionally the resultant mitral regurgitation, especially if both cusps are prolapsing, may be severe and the murmur pansystolic and indistinguishable from that produced by any of the other causes of mitral regurgitation.

Infective endocarditis

Infective endocarditis rarely occurs in the absence of a murmur and most frequently with mild mitral or aortic regurgitation. The condition is notably rare in severe mitral stenosis.

A change in the quality of a previously present mitral systolic murmur may provide a helpful clue when there is uncertainty as to the diagnosis of infective endocarditis. After treatment the healing process with sclerosis may result in increased severity of the valve lesion.

Congenital mitral regurgitation

Congenital mitral regurgitation is usually due to a cleft in the aortic cusp of the valve associated with maldevelopment of the endocardial cushions and a persistent ostium primum in the interatrial septum.

In a patient with signs of an atrial septal defect, a mitral systolic murmur strongly suggests that the defect is of the ostium primum variety and is therefore important in relation to surgical treatment.

Cardiomyopathy

Mitral regurgitation may result from a variety of causes in cardiomyopathy including distortion, papillary muscle dysfunction and cardiac failure.

Trauma

The most frequent cause of traumatic mitral regurgitation is mitral valvotomy. Rarely, rupture of a cusp or chordae results from external trauma.

Left atrial myxoma

Although this condition is less common, it is now readily diagnosable by echocardiography. A fleshy, pedunculated tumour arising from the left atrial wall may prolapse through the mitral valve during diastole producing signs of mitral valve obstruction. Also by distorting and interfering with the closure of the mitral valve during systole it produces mitral regurgitation. The auscultatory signs are therefore those of both mitral stenosis and regurgitation.

TRANSMITTED MURMURS

It has already been emphasised that the murmur of aortic stenosis may be loudest at the apex and thus cause confusion in diagnosis. Despite the classical differences in timing and in quality, when aortic stenosis and mitral regurgitation are both present, differentiation by auscultation may be impossible.

Sometimes in patients with enlargement of the heart a systolic murmur from tricuspid regurgitation is loudest at the apex and may be mistaken for that of mitral regurgitation. In such cases it may be noted that the loudness of the murmur increases during and shortly after a slow, deep inspiration in contrast to the murmur of mitral regurgitation which usually decreases in intensity.

In ventricular septal defect, whether congenital or due to myocardial infarction, the murmur is usually loudest at the left sternal border at about the level of the fourth rib but, if loud, may be well heard at the apex.

In small children differentiation between murmurs due to

a ventricular septal defect, aortic stenosis, and mitral regurgitation may be difficult.

LEFT PARASTERNAL SYSTOLIC MURMURS

A systolic murmur which is loudest at the left sternal border is most likely to be due to one of the causes listed below.

Increased pulmonary blood flow
Obstruction to right ventricular outflow
Ventricular septal defect
Tricuspid regurgitation
Obstruction to left ventricular outflow
Idiopathic

The clinical features of these various conditions are described under the appropriate headings.

If there is other evidence of heart disease in the form of cardiac enlargement or hypertrophy it will be important to establish the cause and, since accuracy in diagnosis is an essential prerequisite for the consideration of surgical treatment, cardiac catheterisation will often be necessary. However, the most likely cause will usually be indicated by clinical examination.

Upper sternal border

The commonest causes are increased pulmonary blood flow or obstruction to right ventricular outflow.

Sometimes only a systolic murmur is present in a patient with patency of the ductus arteriosus, either in infancy when the pulmonary vascular resistance is still relatively high, or in later life if secondary pulmonary hypertension develops.

Midsternal border

The commonest cause of a systolic murmur which is loudest

in the third or fourth intercostal space is a ventricular septal defect and in such cases is often, but not invariably, accompanied by a thrill. The murmur may be pansystolic because, throughout systole, pressure in the left ventricle is greater than that in the right ventricle but can be relatively short if the pulmonary vascular resistance is raised.

A murmur which is loudest in this region may of course be transmitted from elsewhere.

Lower sternal border

A systolic murmur which is loudest at the lower sternal border may be due to tricuspid regurgitation. This may result from organic deformity of the cusps due to rheumatic endocarditis or to dilatation of the valve ring with cardiac failure due to pulmonary hypertension, especially in mitral stenosis. This murmur often increases in intensity during and shortly after deep inspiration (p. 45).

A loud systolic murmur from a neighbouring region may also be audible here.

Isolated 'vibratory' parasternal murmur

A left lower parasternal systolic murmur without any other abnormality to suggest heart disease is a frequent finding in youth and often has a characteristic vibratory quality. In such cases the best term to use is 'idiopathic'.

COMMENT ON TERMINOLOGY

The term 'functional' is often used to signify the presence of a murmur in the absence of any evidence of structural abnormality. However, functional is also frequently used when a murmur from mitral or tricuspid regurgitation is secondary to dilatation of the valve ring rather than to organic disease of the cusps. It is therefore better avoided as an alternative to 'innocent'.

The term 'innocent' is likewise open to objection because it is not always possible to be certain from a single examination that an apparently innocent systolic murmur is not due to mild organic disease, or, of course, that such disease may not in time be progressive. For example a faint aortic systolic murmur may be based on a congenital bicuspid valve which in later life will become calcified and narrow.

Likewise, a faint apical systolic murmur may be due to rheumatic valvitis with slight regurgitation to be followed in due course by mitral stenosis or by infective endocarditis.

Nevertheless, there are occasions when the term 'innocent' is justified, as, for example, when applied to the pulmonary systolic murmur so often present in healthy children or during pregnancy. A similar murmur may be due to increased blood flow from anaemia or thyrotoxicosis.

'*Isolated*' may be used when there is no other evidence of heart disease and '*idiopathic*' when the cause is obscure.

The chief danger is usually that of engendering anxiety when a murmur is found as an isolated anomaly in the absence of other evidence of heart disease. It is very important to avoid this and also the imposition of unwarranted restrictions. Infants and children must be kept under observation and examined at intervals because, at this age, it is often impossible to be certain as to the nature of a systolic murmur.

In young adults it is best to arrange for re-examination after, say, 12 months, but at the same time to give reassurance that no restrictions in activity are indicated and that a normal life can be led in every way.

In older patients an isolated systolic murmur can more readily be ignored, but again it should be remembered that in youth an aortic systolic murmur may signify valve stenosis which does not become of haemodynamic significance until quite late in life, for example after the age of 50. In the elderly, common causes for unimportant systolic murmurs are sclerosis of the aortic valve or calcification of the mitral ring. Papillary muscle dysfunction is another cause of mild mitral regurgitation and its significance is dependent upon that of associated coronary heart disease.

Haemic murmur

The term 'haemic murmur' is best avoided in that it only signifies a murmur associated with a hyperkinetic circulation. In the majority of such cases the murmur is that of increased pulmonary blood flow but, on occasion, with severe anaemia, there may be dilatation of the valve ring with functional mitral regurgitation.

In all cases it is best to state, when possible, the site of origin of the murmur or, when this cannot be ascertained, to use the term 'idiopathic'.

There is no harm in using the term 'isolated' when there is no other abnormality to be found, but in such cases one of the other terms referred to above is usually preferable.

APPROACH TO AN ISOLATED SYSTOLIC MURMUR

An isolated systolic murmur may be due to increased blood flow across a normal valve, to valve disease, to an intra- or extracardiac shunt or to vascular narrowing. Attention should be paid to its site of maximal intensity, radiation, loudness, timing, duration and quality, the effect of changes of posture and respiration, the presence or absence of a thrill, and any abnormality of the heart sounds. An isolated systolic murmur, that is to say with normal heart sounds and in the absence of a thrill, diastolic murmur, cardiac enlargement, hypertrophy or failure, and with a normal X-ray and ECG, can usually be ignored and the patient reassured. Sometimes, as indicated above, a review at intervals is wise. An occasional error may be made by ignoring such a murmur but the risk of this is much less than that of engendering anxiety or imposing unwarranted restrictions.

EXTRACARDIAC MURMURS

Extracardiac murmurs, other than those due to pericarditis, often cause confusion to the inexperienced observer. They may be pericardial or pleuropericardial in origin, even in the absence of inflammation, but from the clinical aspect it is not always possible to be certain as to precise methods of production. They are usually different in quality from murmurs due to heart disease and are often more easy to recognise than to describe. Their importance lies in lack of serious significance.

A *cardiorespiratory murmur* is systolic in time and varies regularly with inspiration. This murmur does not have the characteristics of organic heart disease and is probably due to compression of the expanded lung by the heart during inspiration.

In all such conditions the patient appears well and there is no evidence for any structural abnormality of the heart.

Pericardial friction

A pericardial rub is caused by friction between the visceral and parietal layers and has a characteristic, superficial, scratching quality which, in the appropriate setting, can usually be recognised. It is notoriously variable in situation and in intensity from time to time and even from hour to hour, and hence must be assiduously sought in a patient complaining of acute pain in the chest for which the cause is not obvious.

Precise timing of the components is also variable and the 'rub' may be triphasic, biphasic or monophasic, and sometimes is better heard during inspiration or expiration. Coarse pericardial friction may be palpable.

Pericardial friction may be mistaken for the 'to-and-fro' systolic and diastolic murmurs of aortic valve disease and may be simulated by other extracardiac sounds.

It may be heard in a wide variety of clinical conditions including rheumatic fever, acute myocardial infarction, the post-myocardial infarction syndrome, tuberculosis, rheumatoid arthritis, gout, lupus erythematosus, uraemia, neoplastic invasion, pyogenic infection and after pericardiotomy. Less frequent causes include myxoedema, X-ray therapy, serum sickness, drug hypersensitivity, vaccination, fungal infection, parasitic infection, trauma to the chest wall and penetrating wounds.

DIASTOLIC MURMURS

Classification

Early

Aortic regurgitation
Pulmonary regurgitation

Mid

1. Obstruction
    Mitral stenosis
    Tricuspid stenosis
2. Increased flow
    Mitral
        Mitral regurgitation
        Patent ductus arteriosus
        Ventricular septal defect
    Tricuspid
        Tricuspid regurgitation
        Atrial septal defect

Late (presystolic)

Mitral stenosis
Tricuspid stenosis
Ebstein's Anomaly of the tricuspid valve

Diastolic murmurs fall between the second and first heart sounds and always signify the presence of organic heart disease.

They may be due to:

1. Deformity of the valve cusps
2. Dilatation of the valve ring
3. Increased blood flow.

On the basis of timing they can be classified into three groups:

1. *Early* — beginning with the second sound and due to regurgitant flow through the aortic or pulmonary valve.
2. *Mid* — beginning a short interval after semilunar valve closure (and therefore not precisely in mid-diastole) and due to forward flow through the mitral or tricuspid valve.
3. *Late* — beginning in presystole or from apparent accentuation of a murmur starting earlier in diastole, and dependent on atrial contraction.

EARLY DIASTOLIC MURMURS

In order to understand why diastolic regurgitant murmurs begin with the second sound it is helpful to study the haemodynamics of the cardiac cycle. For the sake of simplicity the left ventricular and aortic pressures and their relationship to aortic regurgitation will be discussed. It must be remembered however that precisely the same reasoning can be applied to the association between right ventricular and pulmonary artery pressures and pulmonary regurgitation.

As the left ventricle relaxes during the latter part of systole its pressure falls below that in the aorta. At this point the aortic valve closes and the aortic component of the second sound occurs. From this point on there exists a pressure difference between aorta and left ventricle which in the presence of an incompetent aortic valve will cause blood to flow from aorta to left ventricle. The regurgitant murmur thus produced will therefore begin with the aortic component of the second sound and will continue for as long as flow is great enough to create an audible murmur. If the leak is small (Fig. 18a), there will still be a large pressure difference between aorta and left ventricle even at the end of diastole so that regurgitant flow will continue throughout diastole producing a long diastolic murmur which diminishes only a little in intensity towards the end of diastole.

In contrast if the defect in the aortic valve is large (Fig. 18b), allowing free regurgitation, the fall in aortic pressure and rise in left ventricular diastolic pressure will be rapid. In extreme cases the pressures may equalise at around 30 to 40 mmHg. The pressure difference between aorta and left ventricle therefore diminishes rapidly as diastole progresses and hence the driving force producing the regurgitant flow will also diminish rapidly. The resultant regurgitant murmur begins as before with aortic closure and although relatively loud initially diminishes rapidly in intensity and may become inaudible well before the end of diastole. This explains not only the early diastolic nature of the murmur but the relatively short, decrescendo character of the diastolic murmur of severe regurgitation.

It will be noted that if the second sound is still normally split, in other words with aortic closure (A_2) preceding pulmonary closure (P_2), the onset of the aortic regurgitant murmur precedes pulmonary closure (Fig. 19a). In severe aortic regurgitation the increased volume of blood to be ejected from left ventricle may result in reversed splitting of the

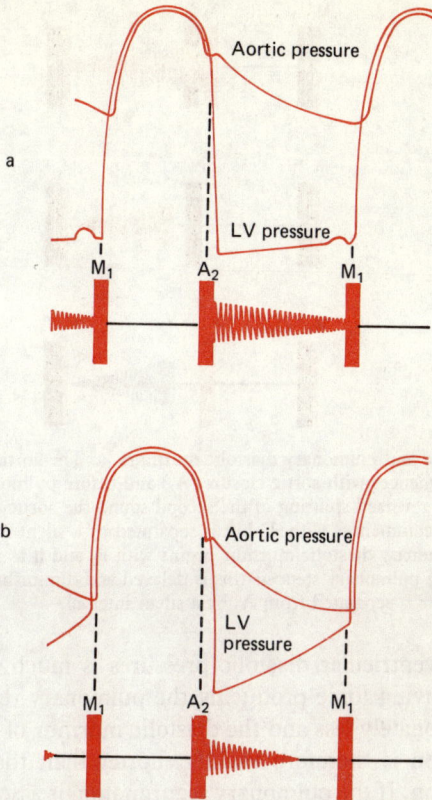

Fig. 18 Aortic early diastolic murmur. The effect of the difference between aortic and left ventricular pressure in diastole on the length of the aortic diastolic murmur is shown in (a) mild and (b) severe aortic regurgitation.

second sound (p. 79). If A_2 is soft or inaudible the onset of the aortic diastolic murmur may be separated from the only audible second sound (P_2) by a short interval (Fig. 19b).

In pulmonary regurgitation, unless severe pulmonary hypertension is present, the difference between pulmonary artery

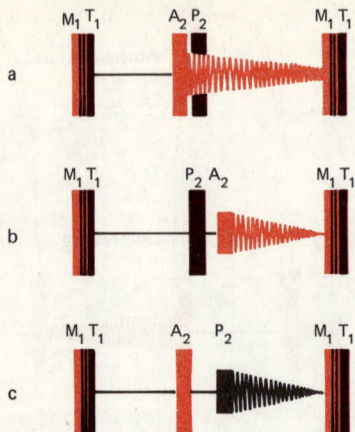

Fig. 19 Aortic and pulmonary diastolic murmurs. a. The aortic diastolic murmur commences with aortic closure (A_2) and before pulmonary closure (P_2). b. With reversed splitting of the second sound the aortic diastolic murmur still commences with A_2 but is separated by a silent interval from P_2. c. A pulmonary diastolic murmur begins with P_2 and if as in accompanying pulmonary stenosis this is delayed and diminished the onset of the murmur is separated from A_2 by a silent interval.

and right ventricular diastolic pressures is much smaller, so that the driving force producing the pulmonary regurgitation is proportionately less and the diastolic murmur of pulmonary regurgitation is therefore usually shorter than that of aortic regurgitation. If the pulmonary regurgitation is associated with pulmonary stenosis and a delayed, soft or absent P_2, the onset of the diastolic murmur may be separated from the only audible component of the second sound (A_2) by an interval (Fig. 19c).

Aortic regurgitation

Aetiology

Aortic regurgitation may arise from deformity or disease of the valve cusps or from dilatation of the valve ring and may be due to congenital or acquired defects.

Congenital: Bicuspid aortic valve
Imperfect closure of valve
Infective endocarditis
Coarctation of the aorta
Aortic stenosis with rigid cusps
Fenestration of the cusps
Marfan's disease
High ventricular septal defect
Aneurysm of sinus of Valsalva
Subvalvar aortic stenosis

Acquired: Rheumatic
Syphilitic
Infective endocarditis
Dissecting aneurysm
Rheumatoid arthritis
Ankylosing spondylitis
Reiter's syndrome
Disseminated lupus erythematosus
Traumatic
Hypertension
Atherosclerosis
Leaking prosthetic valve

The diastolic murmur of aortic regurgitation is usually loudest in the third and fourth intercostal spaces, close to the left sternal border. If loud it may also be heard at the apex, in which case it can usually be appreciated that there is no gap between the second sound and the beginning of the murmur. This is in contrast to the diastolic murmur of mitral stenosis when there is a distinct gap and often a preceding opening snap, as discussed on p. 134.

The murmur of aortic regurgitation is best heard with a diaphragm chest piece and with the patient sitting up or standing and with the breath held in expiration. It is well to remember these points if quiet murmurs are not to be overlooked. The murmur is usually high-pitched and blowing in quality.

If harsh or musical, and especially if heard best to the right rather than to the left of the sternum, causes other than rheumatic fever should be considered. These include rupture of an aortic cusp, infective endocarditis, syphilis, leaking aneurysm of a sinus of Valsalva and rupture of a dissecting aneurysm with dilatation of the valve ring. Occasionally a similar murmur may be heard when there is gross dilatation of the ascending aorta immediately above the valve. Differentiation can usually be made by consideration of associated circumstances.

Although in general a loud murmur will be associated with severe regurgitation, there is no close correlation between these two features. For reasons discussed on p. 126, a loud, rapidly decrescendo murmur is more likely to be associated with severe regurgitation than is a softer murmur occupying the whole of diastole.

With free regurgitation there will be a full, sharply collapsing 'water hammer' pulse and a low diastolic blood pressure with a high systolic pressure and therefore high pulse pressure. Exaggerated arterial pulsations may be obvious in the carotid and other arteries and capillary pulsation in the nail beds or in the retinal vessels. A 'pistol' shot may be heard over a medium-sized vessel, such as the brachial or femoral artery, if the vessel is lightly compressed with the bell of the stethoscope. Nevertheless, severe regurgitation in association with stenosis, may be present without these signs. When accompanied by significant stenosis the brachial and carotid pulses are *bisferiens* rather than collapsing in quality (p. 23). Occasionally a rigid arterial system such as in advanced arteriosclerosis or syphilitic aortitis can produce a misleadingly collapsing pulse with a wide pulse pressure which may result in an over-estimation of the severity of the aortic regurgitation.

The actual *causes of regurgitation* include contraction of the cusps, dilatation of the valve ring, erosion or rupture of a cusp, separation of the commissures and congenital malformation.

Most of these conditions are now amenable to surgical treatment and therefore precision in diagnosis is important.

Aetiology

It is helpful to keep in mind the various conditions which may give rise to aortic regurgitation (p. 129).

The younger the patient the more likely is the defect to be due to congenital malformation.

Rheumatic fever is the most frequent cause, in which case there is often associated mitral disease.

In aortic stenosis the valve is often rigid and the cusps do not come into perfect apposition during diastole so that some degree of regurgitation is frequent, even with severe stenosis.

Infective endocarditis usually affects an already abnormal valve from congenital malformation or rheumatic fever.

Syphilis, although now uncommon, should be remembered in isolated aortic regurgitation, especially in middle-aged and younger men.

A congenital bicuspid valve is a common anomaly but more often gives rise to stenosis than regurgitation.

A high ventricular septal defect of the perimembranous subvalvar (supracristal) type, is situated just below the aortic valve and in consequence a cusp may be unsupported and prolapse into the left ventricle in diastole.

Features of the Marfan syndrome should be sought in cases of obscure aetiology.

Proximal dissection of an aortic aneurysm may be responsible for an early diastolic murmur in a patient with the sudden onset of pain in the chest.

Likewise, the sudden onset of dyspnoea may be due to

rupture of an aneurysm of a sinus of Valsalva. If this is into a right sided cardiac chamber of left atrium a continuous murmur is usual but if into the left ventricle, there may only be a diastolic murmur.

Disorders of connective tissue sometimes also involve the root of the aorta or valve cusps.

Severe systemic hypertension and atherosclerosis of the aorta, which often occur together, are occasional causes for mild aortic regurgitation.

Nowadays a leaking prosthetic valve has become a relatively common cause and may require further operation, often on account of haemolysis.

Pulmonary regurgitation

Aetiology

Congenital causes: Bicuspid valve
Other malformation of cusps
Dilatation of pulmonary artery
Pulmonary stenosis
Pulmonary hypertension

Acquired causes: Pulmonary hypertension
Mitral disease
Pulmonary heart disease
Massive pulmonary embolism
Idiopathic
Surgical treatment for pulmonary stenosis
Miscellaneous rarities
Rheumatic fever, syphilis, infective endo-carditis, carcinoid syndrome and external trauma

An early diastolic murmur from pulmonary regurgitation was first described by Graham–Steell in a patient with severe pulmonary hypertension from mitral stenosis but also occurs in a number of other conditions (p. 132). The murmur is similar in quality to that of aortic regurgitation and likewise audible down the left sternal border. It may be impossible to distinguish the two by auscultation and in patients with rheumatic heart disease the probability as to which valve is at fault must be decided by seeking signs of aortic regurgitation in the peripheral circulation on the one hand and those of pulmonary hypertension on the other. However, the pulmonary diastolic murmur will often become louder on inspiration, whereas the aortic diastolic murmur will remain unchanged or become softer.

Pulmonary hypertension will be indicated by a loud pulmonary component of the second heart sound, by clinical or electro-cardiographic evidence of right ventricular hypertrophy and by radiographic enlargement of the main pulmonary artery and its first two branches. However, it is not possible to diagnose a Graham–Steell murmur with certainty before operation because, in patients with mitral stenosis, associated mild aortic regurgitation, that is without peripheral signs, is frequent. If, following mitral valve surgery, the early diastolic murmur disappears then, in retrospect, the diagnosis can be made with confidence. It is rare in the Western world today to see patients with mitral stenosis accompanied by pulmonary hypertension severe enough to produce pulmonary regurgitation. It is also unusual for mitral stenosis to go unrecognised for long enough to produce this. Many patients will have had previous valvotomies. Statistically therefore a diagnosis of aortic regurgitation in such patients has more chance of being correct.

Pulmonary regurgitation may also occur with gross dilatation of the pulmonary artery from any cause including isolated, idiopathic dilatation.

Pulmonary valve surgery for relief of pulmonary stenosis or correction of Fallot's tetralogy is not frequently followed by pulmonary regurgitation, especially where a hypoplastic main pulmonary artery and valve ring have necessitated insertion of a gusset.

MID-DIASTOLIC MURMURS

A mid-diastolic murmur may be heard in mitral or tricuspid stenosis or with increased flow across the valve without stenosis.

Actually 'mid' is not strictly accurate with regard to valvar stenosis because the murmur starts a short interval after the second sound immediately following the opening snap of the mitral or tricuspid valve. However, merely to call it a mitral or tricuspid diastolic murmur does not distinguish it from a presystolic murmur and the term is therefore convenient.

The reason for the mid-diastolic nature of diastolic forward-flow murmurs becomes apparent when the associated changes in atrial and ventricular pressures during diastole are examined. For the sake of simplicity only the left heart pressures in relationship to mitral stenosis will be considered but it must be remembered that precisely the same relationships exist between right heart pressures and tricuspid stenosis.

As the left ventricle (LV) relaxes towards the end of systole its pressure falls below that of the aorta. The aortic component of the second sound (A_2) occurs with closure of the aortic valve. The LV pressure is still however above that in the left atrium (LA) so that the mitral valve is still closed. There is thus a brief period after A_2, during which blood is neither leaving nor entering the LV (the isovolumic relaxation phase). When the LV pressure falls below that in the LA the mitral valve opens and when the opening is at its widest the opening snap occurs (Fig. 20a). If the LA pressure or more precisely the v wave of LA pressure is raised the time taken for LV pressure to fall from the point at which A_2 occurred to the point of mitral valve opening will be shorter (Fig. 20b) thus

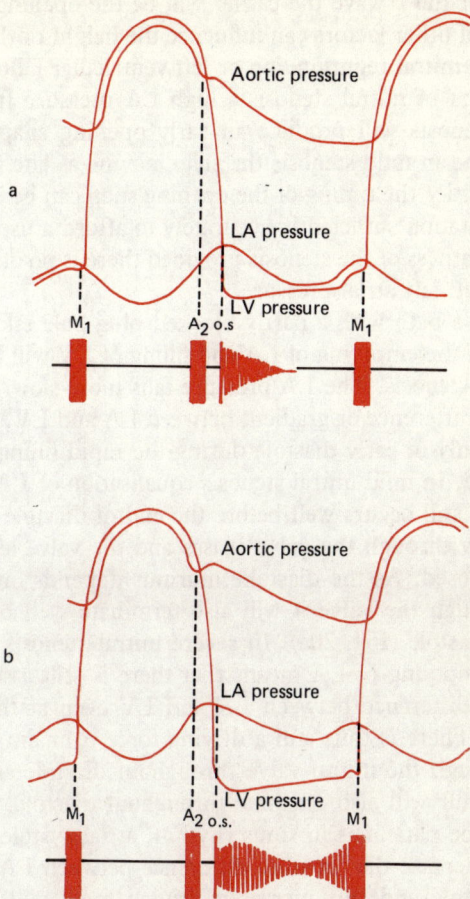

Fig. 20 Mitral mid-diastolic murmur. The timing of the heart sounds, opening snap and murmur is shown in relation to the changes in left heart pressures. The effect of the raised left atrial pressure and the pressure difference between LA and LV in diastole on the earliness of the opening snap and the length of the mitral diastolic murmur is shown in (a) mild and (b) severe mitral stenosis.

the higher the v wave the earlier will be the opening snap. A number of other factors can influence the height of the v wave including mitral regurgitation or left ventricular failure but in the context of mitral stenosis a high LA pressure from tight mitral stenosis will produce an early opening snap (around 0.06 s) and in mild stenosis the snap may be as late as 0.12 s. With practice the timing of the opening snap can be estimated by auscultation sufficiently accurately to afford a useful guide to the tightness of the stenosis provided there is no other cause for a raised left atrial pressure.

Just as a bath with a partly blocked plug-hole takes longer to empty, the emptying of LA and filling of LV will be slower in mitral stenosis. The LA pressure falls more slowly and the pressure difference or gradient between LA and LV, normally present only in early diastole during the rapid filling phase is prolonged. In mild mitral stenosis equalisation of LA and LV pressures still occurs well before the end of diastole at which point flow through the valve ceases and the valve leaflets are loosely closed. As the diastolic murmur depends on forward flow through the valve it will also terminate well before the end of diastole (Fig. 20a). In severe mitral stenosis the slow rate of emptying of LA means that there is still a significant pressure difference between LA and LV even at the end of diastole. There is thus still a driving force to maintain blood flow through the mitral valve throughout diastole and hence the murmur will also continue throughout diastole. Furthermore if the patient is in sinus rhythm, atrial systole will still further increase the pressure difference between LA and LV in presystole and this increased driving force will result in increased flow through the mitral valve and a presystolic accentuation of the murmur (Fig. 20b).

In summary, tight mitral stenosis will be associated with an early opening snap and a full length mitral diastolic murmur whereas in mild mitral stenosis the opening snap will be late and the diastolic murmur short. Mitral diastolic flow murmurs not associated with stenosis of the valve will also be short because early equalisation of LA and LV pressure means that forward-flow through the mitral valves ceases early.

The causes are listed in the table on page 141.

Mitral stenosis

The cardinal sign of mitral stenosis is a long, rumbling, diastolic murmur, loudest at, or localised to, the apex. If, as is so often the case, atrial fibrillation is present, there will be no presystolic accentuation.

This murmur is best heard or may only be heard if the patient is lying down and turned towards the left side, or if blood flow is increased by exercise. These manoeuvres should therefore be part of the routine examination of any patient suspected of having mitral disease.

The *classical* signs of mitral stenosis are a loud, slapping, first heart sound preceded by a crescendo presystolic murmur and an opening snap followed by a rumbling, mid-diastolic murmur. This cadence gives rise to the onomatopoeic 'ffout ta ta rrou' first described by Duroziez (Fig. 21).

The first or presystolic element of this sequence occurs late in ventricular diastole, synchronous with the forceful passage of blood into the ventricle produced by atrial systole. This presystolic accentuation is only heard in patients with sinus rhythm and disappears with the onset of fibrillation. It is

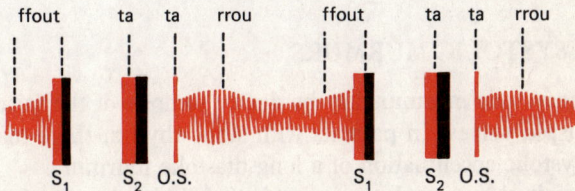

incorrect to say that the *presystolic murmur* disappears because the diastolic murmur may continue up to the first sound and it is only the crescendo accentuation which is absent in atrial fibrillation.

It used to be thought that a mitral diastolic murmur at the apex was diagnostic of obstruction but, with the increased precision in auscultation which came with phonocardiography, and, in particular, the stimulus to careful auscultation brought by the advent of cardiac surgery, it was recognised that a murmur, similar in time but different in origin, may occur in patients with increased blood flow across the valve. The advent of echocardiography provided further confirmation of this. Such conditions include mitral regurgitation, ventricular septal defect and patent ductus arteriosus, and are discussed below.

Tricuspid stenosis

The diastolic murmur of tricuspid stenosis is best heard to the left of the lower sternal border or nearer the apex and becomes loudest during, and immediately after, deep inspiration owing to increased right atrial filling from the great veins. It is not usually rumbling in quality as is the diastolic murmur of mitral stenosis. The opening snap of tricuspid stenosis is usually earlier than that of mitral stenosis but is difficult or impossible to distinguish. As tricuspid stenosis is usually associated with mitral stenosis the inspiratory nature of the tricuspid diastolic murmur may be the only auscultatory clue to its presence.

PRESYSTOLIC MURMURS

A presystolic murmur may be due to stenosis of the mitral or tricuspid valves. In patients with sinus rhythm there may be presystolic accentuation of a long diastolic murmur.

A mitral presystolic murmur is usually loudest precisely at the apex and may be accompanied by a short thrill. An isolated presystolic murmur, that is without an associated mid-diastolic murmur, is only found in the early or mild stages of mitral stenosis.

A presystolic murmur, similar in quality to mitral stenosis, may be heard with tricuspid stenosis. This possibility should always be considered in patients with signs of mitral disease, especially if the presystolic murmur is very clear, well heard towards the sternum and is louder in deep inspiration, which increases blood flow across the tricuspid valve. In such cases there is likely to be a prominent 'a' wave in the jugular venous pulse and a peaked 'P' wave in the electrocardiogram.

Austin Flint murmur

Austin Flint originally described a presystolic murmur in a patient with aortic regurgitation but without mitral disease. However, it has become customary in such cases to use this eponym for any apical diastolic murmur simulating that of mitral stenosis but without other evidence for it.

In patients with aortic regurgitation of non-rheumatic aetiology, such as syphilis, this murmur may be diagnosed with reasonable confidence, but in those with rheumatic heart disease it is usually necessary to carry out echocardiography to confirm a normal mitral valve before arriving at a diagnosis of an Austin Flint murmur.

In the past a number of different theories have been advanced to explain this murmur. They include the production of diastolic mitral regurgitation from reversal of the LV–LA gradient with a resultant backward flow through the valve. Such diastolic regurgitation can be demonstrated not infrequently during left ventricular cineangiography when diastole is unduly prolonged such as during the compensatory pause following a ventricular ectopic beat. However, this is often seen in patients without aortic regurgitation, with a normal mitral valve and no murmurs. With the advent of echocardiography it was noted that characteristic vibrations of the anterior leaflet of the mitral valve occur in association with aortic regurgitation and this mechanism was advanced as the cause of the murmur. However the frequency of these vibrations is related to that of an early diastolic murmur and is too high to explain the low frequency Austin Flint murmur. It has now been demonstrated beyond reasonable doubt that the mechanism of the Austin Flint murmur is forward-flow through the mitral valve when this is in the act of closing as a result of the build up of left ventricular pressure because of the aortic regurgitation. When a high end-diastolic pressure in severe aortic regurgitation results in premature closure of the mitral valve before the end of diastole the late diastolic phase of the Austin Flint murmur is also eliminated.

The same mechanism of antegrade flow across a closing mitral valve has been shown to operate in other conditions associated with a mitral diastolic murmur in the absence of mitral stenosis. For example the short mitral diastolic murmur associated with severe mitral regurgitation begins with a third sound *after* the phase of rapid filling which is relatively silent but coincides with the time at which the mitral valve is beginning to close due to the steeply rising left ventricular diastolic pressure.

Recent studies have demonstrated that while the presystolic murmur of mitral stenosis is initiated by *atrial* systole, the final characteristic crescendo phase of the murmur which culminates in the loud first sound depends on ventricular systole which results in rapid closure of the valve while antegrade flow across it is still in progress. This mechanism also explains the persistence of the latter part of the presystolic crescendo observed occasionally in patients with atrial fibrillation. Nevertheless it would be wise for the student to confine his diagnosis of a presystolic murmur to those patients in whom sinus rhythm is present in order to avoid a controversial confrontation with the examiner!

APICAL DIASTOLIC MURMURS

Aetiology

Mitral stenosis
Increased mitral flow
  Mitral regurgitation
  Ventricular septal defect
  Patent ductus arteriosus

Rheumatic fever (Carey Coombs murmur)
Austin Flint murmur
Transmission of other murmurs
  Aortic regurgitation
  Pulmonary regurgitation
  Tricuspid stenosis
  Increased tricuspid flow
Coarctation of the aorta

An apical diastolic murmur is most frequently due to mitral stenosis but may also occur in a number of other conditions including increased blood flow across the mitral valve and transmission from other areas.

In the acute stage of rheumatic fever there may be a transient, short, diastolic murmur, as first described by Carey Coombs. It is probably due to oedema of the cusps.

In severe mitral regurgitation, owing to increased blood flow across the valve, there is often a decrescendo murmur in mid-diastole which begins abruptly and usually after a third heart sound.

In ventricular septal defect and patency of the ductus arteriosus there may be a similar diastolic murmur from increased flow together with characteristic signs of the primary condition.

The murmurs of aortic and pulmonary regurgitation begin early after the second sound and are usually loudest at the left sternal border but may be well heard at the apex.

In isolated aortic regurgitation there may be a mitral diastolic murmur, as first described by Austin Flint.

In tricuspid stenosis and with increased tricuspid flow, as from a large atrial septal defect with considerable cardiac enlargement, the diastolic murmur may be loudest at the apex.

In coarctation of the aorta an apical diastolic murmur is occasionally present. No satisfactory explanation for this has yet been advanced.

CONTINUOUS MURMURS

Aortopulmonary shunts

Patent ductus arteriosus
Aortopulmonary window
Palliative surgery for cyanotic congenital heart disease

Arterial constriction

Coarctation
Carotid or renal artery stenosis
Pulmonary artery branch stenosis
Bronchopulmonary arterial anastomoses
Collateral arteries

Arteriovenous fistulae

Pulmonary
Systemic
Congenital
Acquired
  Surgical
  Ruptured Sinus of Valsalva
  Trauma
  Paget's disease
  Vascular tumours or malformations

Excessive blood flow

Thyrotoxicosis
Pregnancy (uterine souffle)
Lactation (mammary souffle)

Venous constriction

Venous hum
Anomalous pulmonary venous connection

Constriction between two chambers

Cor triatriatum

A continuous murmur is one which begins in systole and continues through the second sound into diastole. When used in this strict sense the term is correct. It is however sometimes used to mean that the murmur never stops and is continuous throughout systole and diastole. While undoubtedly some murmurs are continuous in this sense it is by no means true of all those to which this term is applied.

A continuous murmur is produced by blood flowing through a tube or from one chamber to another via a constriction which is not a valve. It follows that for flow to take place there must be a pressure difference between the two ends of a tube or between two chambers. The magnitude of this pressure difference will determine the character of the murmur.

The chief causes of a continuous murmur are listed in the table.

Patent ductus arteriosus is by far the most frequent *pathological* cause and was first described by Dr Gibson of Edinburgh. It is often truly continuous, when it has a characteristic 'machinery-like' quality with accentuation in late systole when the gradient is greatest and is loudest in the second left intercostal space. In contrast with a venous hum it is usually loudest on expiration, when the pulmonary artery pressure is lowest.

In infancy only a systolic murmur may be present because of the relatively high pressure in the pulmonary artery. Likewise, if in later years pulmonary hypertension develops, the diastolic part of the murmur shortens and finally disappears. Later the systolic part may also be abbreviated and in some cases, when the pressures are balanced no murmur may be audible.

An *aortopulmonary window* just above the valves is a similar but much rarer condition and more liable to be associated with pulmonary hypertension. It cannot be distinguished with certainty clinically but can usually be identified by 2-D echocardiography.

The reasons for the varied character of these murmurs can be better understood if they are considered in relation to the pressure difference which exists across the constriction producing the murmur and how this changes from moment to moment with systole and diastole.

The aorta and pulmonary artery can be regarded as opposite ends of a tube through which blood is flowing via a constriction (the patent ductus). If a small patent ductus produces a narrow constriction between aorta and pulmonary artery there will be a large pressure difference between aorta and pulmonary artery at all times. This difference will be greatest at the systolic peak of the pressure wave and least at the diastolic trough. The flow through the constriction (ductus) will vary in proportion to this pressure difference and hence the murmur will wax and wane. As there is at all times a pressure difference between the two ends of the tube flow will occur continuously across the constriction and thus the murmur will also be continuous, loudest at the peak of the pressure wave and becoming softer as the pressure difference falls in diastole (Fig. 22a).

If however the patent ductus is large the constriction it produces is correspondingly mild and allows much freer transmission of the aortic pressure wave through to the pulmonary

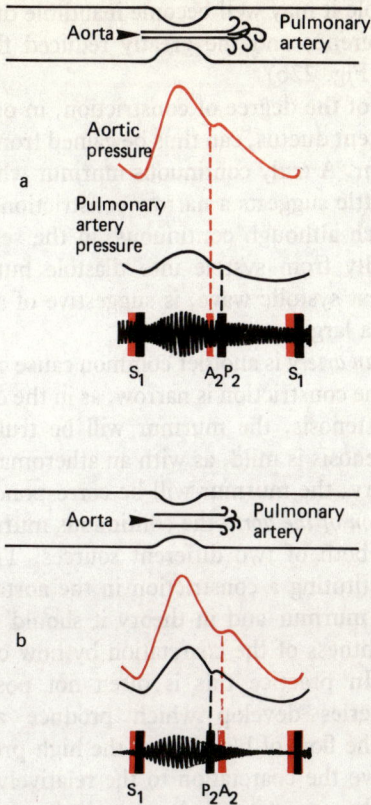

Fig. 22 Continuous murmur of patent ductus arteriosus. The effect of the changing pressure differences between aorta and pulmonary artery on the character of the continuous murmur are shown in (a) a small and (b) a large patent ductus. In a small ductus a large pressure difference is maintained in both systole and diastole and the murmur is truly continuous. In the large ductus the pressure difference becomes small and the murmur soft or absent.

artery. Thus, while there is still a significant pressure difference at the systolic peak of the wave this becomes markedly reduced at the diastolic trough. The resultant murmur will still be loud at the peak of systole but will become rapidly softer until in diastole it may well become inaudible due to the small pressure difference and the greatly reduced flow across the constriction (Fig. 22b).

Some idea of the degree of constriction, in other words the size of the patent ductus, can thus be gained from the character of the murmur. A truly continuous murmur which waxes and wanes very little suggests a narrow constriction. Conversely a murmur which although continuous, in the sense of spilling uninterruptedly from systole into diastole but petering out before the next systolic wave, is suggestive of a much milder constriction (a larger patent ductus).

Stenosis of an artery is another common cause of a continuous murmur. If the constriction is narrow, as in the case of a severe renal artery stenosis, the murmur will be truly continuous. Where the stenosis is mild, as with an atheromatous plaque in a carotid artery, the murmur will be correspondingly short.

In *coarctation of the aorta* the continuous murmur may arise from one or both of two different sources. The coarctation itself by constituting a constriction in the aorta will produce a continuous murmur and in theory it should be possible to assess the tightness of the coarctation by how continuous the murmur is. In practice this is often not possible because collateral arteries develop which produce an alternative pathway for the flow of blood from the high pressure zone in the aorta above the coarctation to the relatively low pressure zone below the coarctation. As these collaterals themselves represent quite a marked constriction between these zones they will also give rise to a continuous murmur which may mask that from the coarctation itself. Sometimes the collateral murmurs can be reduced or obliterated by pressure over the appropriate vessels between the scapulae but often this is not possible.

Continuous murmurs may also occur from bronchial arterial collateral vessels in pulmonary atresia, from pulmonary arterial branch stenosis and rarely from pulmonary embolism with partial occlusion of the vessel.

Continuous arterial murmurs from excessive blood flow may be heard over a hyperactive thyroid gland in thyrotoxicosis and occasionally a mammary souffle may be heard over the lactating breast.

A *venous hum* is a continuous murmur which may be heard quite commonly at the root of the neck and sometimes in the upper chest in children and occasionally in young adults. It is again due to constriction, but in a vein which may be compressed by one of the surrounding structures in the neck such as a ligamentous band or even by a well developed platysma muscle. Unlike the continuous murmur of arterial stenosis it is often loudest in diastole when the venous blood flow towards the heart is increased. For the same reason it usually increases during inspiration. It is often loudest on one side of the neck or other and varies markedly with posture. The simplest test for a venous hum is to obliterate the vein or veins producing the hum by pressure with the finger over the root of the neck on the side of the murmur, which will then disappear or become much softer. Removal of this pressure results in an immediate increase in the loudness of the murmur. A similar accentuation can be produced by turning the head away from the side where the murmur is loudest thereby increasing the compression effect by surrounding structures. Conversely, relaxing the tissues by turning the head to the side of the murmur causes it to diminish or even disappear. If heard below the clavicle the venous hum may simulate a patent ductus and it is therefore important to carry out the procedures outlined above in order to distinguish between the two. Occasionally in a child both may be present. The importance of a venous hum, which is itself a completely innocent condition, is that it may be misinterpreted for some other continuous murmur of pathological significance.

Arteriovenous fistulae may be congenital or acquired. They are sometimes due to surgical treatment as in the creation of an arteriovenous shunt for renal haemodialysis. Similar shunts may be carried out not between an artery and vein but between an artery and the lower pressure pulmonary artery for certain forms of cyanotic congenital heart disease. This deliberate creation of a shunt to increase the blood supply to the lungs often results in a very loud and widely conducted continuous murmur.

The murmur associated with a pulmonary arteriovenous fistula is usually mainly systolic but may occasionally be truly continuous. Where the fistula is large or multiple there may also be central cyanosis and clubbing of the fingers.

A high *ventricular septal defect* may result in an aortic cusp being unsupported with consequent aortic regurgitation. In such cases the murmur is almost continuous, but in the more frequent combination of aortic stenosis and regurgitation there is a distinct, if slight, gap and the murmur is more appropriately described as being 'to and fro' in quality.

There are numerous causes of a continuous murmur and accurace of diagnosis is important because of the wide variation in clinical significance and in differing treatment. However, it will be appreciated that if due consideration is given to all the associated clinical, radiographic, electrocardiographic and echocardiographic features, errors should be uncommon and the indications for specialised investigation will usually be clear.

5

Summaries of clinical features of commonest disorders

The following summaries describe the classical clinical features of fairly severe lesions, but it will be appreciated that all grades of severity may occur and often combinations of lesions.

ACUTE MYOCARDIAL INFARCTION

It would be inappropriate here to describe in detail the clinical manifestations of acute myocardial infarction and its complications, but certain bedside observations in addition to auscultation may be of critical importance, especially in the absence of facilities for monitoring. Early recognition and appropriate management may be life-saving.

The onset of myocardial infarction is usually sudden with collapse, chest pain or dyspnoea.

Cardiac pain may be simulated by various conditions including:

Acute pericarditis.
Chronic benign perimyocarditis.
Massive pulmonary embolism.
Dissecting aneurysm of the aorta.
Oesophageal and upper abdominal disorders.
Skeletal conditions involving the lower cervical and upper thoracic spine.

Sudden death is frequent and often the first manifestation of coronary heart disease. The commonest cause is ventricular fibrillation.

Asystole may be due to pump failure or conduction disturbance.

Dyspnoea from pulmonary venous congestion or oedema is due to left ventricular failure. This may be indicated by crepitations, but routine radiography has shown that pulmonary oedema may be present without abnormal signs in the lungs.

The signs of *shock* are due to a low cardiac output with hypotension and compensatory vasoconstriction. They include a cold clammy skin with a rapid thready pulse and often apathy, restlessness and mental confusion.

Gallop rhythm, especially from the addition of a presystolic (atrial) sound, is commonly present and may be palpable, especially if the patient is turned on to the left side.

Reversed splitting of the second sound may be present due to impaired left ventricular function and may be transient, occurring during an anginal attack and returning to normal with relief of the pain. Very wide reversed splitting or very wide normal splitting suggest left or right bundle branch block respectively.

The most frequent *arrhythmias* are ventricular extrasystoles, ventricular tachycardia, ventricular fibrillation, atrial fibrillation and supraventricular tachycardia but there is no reliable clinical way of diagnosing these conditions. An ECG is essential.

Sinus bradycardia may be present especially if the patient has been receiving beta-receptor blocking drugs.

A *pericardial rub* is often heard during the first 48 hours following myocardial infarction but when occurring later, especially when accompanied by pericardial pain, suggests a post-myocardial infarction syndrome (Dressler's syndrome).

Acute mitral regurgitation is indicated by the sudden development of an apical pansystolic murmur accompanied by signs of left ventricular failure and by pulmonary venous congestion or pulmonary oedema on the chest X-ray. This may be due to ruptured chordae or papillary muscle.

Rupture of the interventricular septum is indicated by the development of a pansystolic murmur, maximal at the left sternal edge, accompanied by signs of left and frequently right ventricular failure and by pulmonary oedema and plethora on the chest X-ray. The distinction between acute mitral regurgitation and ruptured interventricular septum although theoretically clear-cut is in practice often difficult; 2-D echocardiography is invaluable in making the correct diagnosis.

Congestive failure is used for want of a better term and indicates the familiar clinical picture of peripheral oedema, a raised jugular venous pressure and engorgement of the liver, but pulmonary oedema is also 'congestive'. In the present context it is usually secondary to left ventricular failure.

Massive pulmonary embolism is characterised by the sudden onset of respiratory distress with hyperventilation, cyanosis and anxiety. Sometimes true anginal pain is present from myocardial ischaemia due to the reduced coronary blood flow secondary to low cardiac output. Signs of acute right heart failure, with elevation of jugular venous pressure and a right ventricular gallop are present. Lesser degrees of embolism may be suggested by the appearance of pulmonary infarction which do not have time to develop in massive embolism. There are pleuritic pain and haemoptysis together with radiographic evidence of pulmonary infarction.

Right ventricular infarction is also often characterised by acute right heart failure with similar physical signs to those of the acute right heart failure accompanying massive pulmonary embolism. The diagnosis should be suspected when acute right heart failure occurs in a patient with ECG evidence of an inferior or posterior wall infarction.

Abnormal cardiac systolic pulsation in the acute stage of myocardial infarction is sometimes present. The later development of a similar pulsation may be due to *left ventricular aneurysm*. Clinical diagnosis is however unreliable and specialised diagnostic procedures such as echocardiography, radioisotope studies or angiocardiography may be necessary.

Systemic embolism may result from thrombus formation on the ventricular endocardium.

MASSIVE PULMONARY EMBOLISM

The symptoms of massive pulmonary embolism develop suddenly and are mainly due to circulatory obstruction with a fall in cardiac output. Pulmonary infarction may or may not follow.

Often there is a suggestive clinical setting for its development such as phlebothrombosis, the onset of an arrhythmia, a recent operation or pregnancy, unaccustomed bedrest, especially for some debilitating disease, or cardiac failure. In females, the contraceptive pill is an important but rare predisposing factor.

The characteristic features are acute respiratory distress with anxiety, hyperpnoea and a rapid pulse of small volume. Cyanosis may be intense. Sometimes there is pain from myocardial ischaemia but more often a sensation of oppression in the chest.

The jugular venous pressure is raised and the systemic arterial pressure falls. A right ventricular, right atrial or summation gallop is usually present indicating acute right heart failure.

The pulmonary component of the second heart sound may be delayed due to prolongation of right ventricular ejection by increased resistance to outflow and impaired right ventricular function. Signs of pulmonary hypertension are never present unless this was already in existence before the current embolus, for example from a previous embolus.

Occasionally a tricuspid systolic murmur develops.

In severe cases there may be loss of consciousness or the clinical picture of shock, the patient becoming pale, cold and clammy with a weak thready pulse.

Usually there is considerable apprehension and a sensation of impending disaster which is often fulfilled.

Retrosternal pain with the clinical picture of shock may lead to an erroneous diagnosis of myocardial infarction. Conversely, right ventricular myocardial infarction may closely mimic massive pulmonary embolism.

The signs of pulmonary infarction, which may develop later if the patient survives, include pleuritic pain, fever and haemoptysis, but the latter symptom is often absent. Jaundice may follow, due to the breaking down of haemoglobin, in which case urobilinogen will be present in the urine. Pleural friction may be heard and an effusion sometimes develops.

PULMONARY HYPERTENSION

Pulmonary hypertension is suggested by a loud pulmonary component of the second heart sound, palpable pulmonary valve closure, and evidence of right ventricular (RV) hypertrophy. However, there is no close relationship between the degree of pulmonary hypertension (PHT) and the loudness of the second sound.

There may be physical signs of various forms of congenital or acquired heart disease but occasionally the condition may be present without obvious cause (primary pulmonary hypertension).

Other signs include a presystolic gallop rhythm from atrial contraction against increased right ventricular filling resistance, a pulmonary systolic murmur and ejection click and an early diastolic murmur from pulmonary regurgitation. In advanced cases with cardiac failure there may be a third heart sound from right ventricular failure and a pansystolic murmur from functional tricuspid regurgitation. In addition, the pulse may be of small volume with peripheral cyanosis from a low cardiac output.

The detection of PHT is of importance in all cases in which it is present because it indicates the necessity for establishing a precise diagnosis of the underlying cause with a view to appropriate treatment. This may require radiography, electrocardiography, echocardiography and sometimes more elaborate laboratory methods. Likewise, in a negative sense, the *absence* of PHT in a patient with heart disease liable to be associated with it is reassuring, and will often obviate the need for more elaborate methods of investigation.

Congenital conditions are mainly those with a left to right shunt and the principal acquired causes are mitral disease, left ventricular failure, chronic pulmonary disease and massive or recurrent pulmonary embolism.

CARDIAC COMPRESSION

Compression of the heart may result from pericardial fluid or constrictive pericarditis.

The term cardiac tamponade signifies acute compression by an increase in intrapericardial pressure due to haemorrhage or effusion.

The haemodynamic effects of compression are impairment of diastolic filling and consequently of myocardial contraction. As a result stroke volume is reduced and, above a critical level of intrapericardial pressure, the cardiac output falls.

Cardiac tamponade

The amount of fluid which must accumulate before haemodynamic effects are noticeable depends on its rate of formation and the distensibility of the pericardial sac. A large effusion may accumulate slowly with no more than a slight rise in jugular venous pressure. On the other hand acute tamponade may result from a small effusion of rapid development. The situation is clearly an emergency one with the patient distressed, dyspnoeic, apprehensive and complaining of a feeling of oppression in the chest and not actual pain. The most favoured posture is sitting forward with elbows supported, but true orthopnoea is absent.

The principal signs are due to a fall in cardiac output and in systemic arterial pressure with a compensatory rise in systemic venous pressure and tachycardia.

The deep neck veins are engorged with exaggerated pulsation and there may be a paradoxical increase in venous pressure during inspiration, that is to say, the reverse of normal. The radial pulse is rapid and of low volume and characteristically pulsus paradoxus is present, that is to say, there is a significant fall in volume during inspiration (p. 9). Peripheral cyanosis may be present but there is no oedema.

The characteristic cardiac signs are in effect negative ones, that is to say, there may be no evidence of heart disease in the form of cardiac enlargement or hypertrophy and no abnormal sounds or murmurs. There may be muffling or damping of the heart sounds.

Accurate diagnosis is important because pericardial paracentesis may be life saving. Removal of only a few ml of fluid may be followed by dramatic relief.

Aetiological factors to be considered include tuberculosis, viral infection, neoplasm and haemorrhage from trauma, dissecting aneurysm, or after cardiac surgery. Other causes of pericarditis are unlikely to result in acute compression.

BEDSIDE APPROACH TO TACHYCARDIA OR DYSRHYTHMIAS

Although in practice a brief history will first be taken, when the problem is an acute arrhythmia or defect of conduction this aspect will necessarily be limited. However, enquiry should be made as to whether the patient is being treated with digitalis or oral diuretics or, in the case of a conduction defect, with a beta-adrenergic receptor blocking drug and whether there have been previous similar attacks.

The brachial pulse should be felt for rate and rhythm and the jugular venous pulse inspected for atrial waves which may be irregular or more rapid than ventricular waves and for cannon waves which indicate AV dissociation or AV junctional (nodal) rhythm. Cannon waves with bradycardia suggest complete heart block and with tachycardia a ventricular arrhythmia.

Auscultation will confirm rate and rhythm and reveal any pulse deficit, and there may be signs of valve disease. Variation in the intensity of the first heart sound, if not due to atrial fibrillation, suggests AV dissociation.

Palpation of the chest wall may reveal evidence of heart disease in the form of cardiac enlargement or hypertrophy or a thrill.

Carotid sinus massage may terminate an attack of atrial tachycardia, will have no effect on ventricular tachycardia and may temporarily slow the ventricular rate in atrial flutter.

Clinical recognition of many arrhythmias is unreliable or impossible and early electrocardiographic confirmation is essential.

Extrasystoles

Ventricular extrasystoles are characterised by a regular rhythm which is interrupted by premature beats followed by relatively long (compensatory) pauses. The following beat is large and forceful. Atrial systoles may not be followed by a compensatory pause. If multiple extrasystoles are present the condition may simulate atrial fibrillation. Extrasystoles, depending on their cause, may increase or become less frequent or even disappear with exercise. The heart sounds vary in intensity with the duration of the preceding diastole. Ventricular extra-systoles occurring against a background of atrial fibrillation, may be impossible to detect clinically.

Occasional extrasystoles are very common in healthy individuals but may be the cause of palpitation.

They may also be associated with any form of heart disease and usually their significance is entirely that of the severity of the underlying condition. However, in acute myocardial infarction, they may precede a more serious arrhythmia even in relatively mild cases as judged by the severity of myocardial damage.

Atrial fibrillation

Atrial fibrillation should be suspected when the heart beat and radial pulse are totally irregular in time and force.

The condition must be distinguished from multiple extrasystoles and from atrial flutter or tachycardia with varying block.

It may be difficult to be certain of the diagnosis, especially if the ventricular rate is relatively slow, or impossible if there is associated heart block.

Owing to the irregular duration of cardiac cycles the intensity of heart sounds and the duration of murmurs vary from beat to beat.

The most frequent causes of fibrillation should be kept in mind and confirmatory signs sought. These include rheumatic heart disease, coronary heart disease, thyrotoxicosis, myocarditis and cardiomyopathy, constrictive pericarditis and neoplastic invasion. In acute conditions it may result from myocardial infarction, massive pulmonary embolism, thoracotomy, external trauma, electrocution and other rarities. Transient attacks may be precipitated by emotional stimuli or other causes for catecholamine secretion.

It may also occur without obvious cause as an isolated anomaly and persistent or recur over many years.

Atrial flutter

Atrial flutter should be suspected if the heart rate is about 160/minute and flutter waves can be seen in the jugular venous pulse, or if there is temporary ventricular slowing with carotid sinus pressure.

The ventricular rate may be regular or, if there is varying AV block, irregular.

The aetiology of flutter is much the same as for atrial fibrillation but the condition is less frequent.

Atrial and nodal tachycardia

Regular atrial or nodal tachycardia is usually at a rate of about 160–200/minute and most frequently occurs in the absence of any other detectable abnormality but may be a complication of heart disease. It is a common manifestation of digitalis toxicity, especially occurring in a patient previously in atrial fibrillation. In nodal tchycardia contraction of the right atrium in ventricular systole may produce regular 'cannon waves' in the jugular venous pulse.

Atrial tchycardia can often be terminated by carotid sinus massage.

Ventricular tachycardia

Ventricular tachycardia is due to the rapid discharge of an ectopic focus in one or other ventricle. There is no reliable clinical method of diagnosis.

Carotid sinus massage has no effect on this dysrhythmia.

MITRAL STENOSIS

The classical signs are a loud first sound, opening snap and rumbling diastolic murmur with presystolic accentuation if the patients is in sinus rhythm. However, these signs are often modified by complicating factors including sclerosis and calcification of the cusps, a high pulmonary vascular resistance with consequent low blood flow, and other valve defects. In addition a loud first heart sound may be palpable as a tapping impulse, and the murmur is sometimes associated with a corresponding thrill.

In general, the longer the diastolic murmur and the earlier the opening snap the greater the severity of stenosis but there are exceptions and with a low cardiac output the murmur may become short or even disappear. In mild stenosis there may be only a short murmur and a late opening snap. An apical systolic murmur is often present from an associated regurgitant jet or there may be a transmitted murmur here from aortic stenosis or tricuspid regurgitation.

If pulmonary hypertension is present there may be accentuation of the pulmonary component of the second sound and a right ventricular thrust from hypertrophy.

Right ventricular hypertrophy suggests pulmonary hypertension from dominant stenosis. Left ventricular hypertrophy, unless due to associated aortic valve disease or systemic hypertension, suggests dominant regurgitation.

MITRAL REGURGITATION

The characteristic sign of mitral regurgitation is a blowing, apical pansystolic murmur which can be heard towards the left axilla and often as far as the left lung base. The apex beat will be left ventricular and hyperkinetic in character. If regurgitation is severe the first heart sound will be faint or absent and there will be a third heart sound early in diastole near the end of the phase of rapid ventricular filling, and often also a short, decrescendo, diastolic murmur due to increased blood flow from atrium to ventricle. In some forms of mitral regurgitation for example that due to mitral valve prolapse, the systolic murmur occurs late in systole.

MITRAL STENOSIS AND REGURGITATION

Rheumatic endocarditis often results in fusion and sclerosis of the cusps, which cannot come into apposition in systole, with the production of stenosis and regurgitation. In such cases the signs of these two valve defects will be combined.

The differentiation of dominant stenosis or regurgitation can often be made by consideration of all the clinical findings together with radiography and electrocardiography, but in cases of doubt cardiac catheterisation and left ventricular angiocardiography are necessary. Echocardiography is not of great value in quantitating the severity of mitral regurgitation.

AORTIC STENOSIS

The characteristic sign of aortic stenosis is a harsh, systolic ejection murmur which is audible over the upper sternum and to its left, and often down the left sternal border and at the apex. Occasionally it is loudest at the apex and may cause difficulty in differentiation from the murmur of mitral regurgitation or a transmitted murmur from elsewhere. Classically, the murmur is maximal in midsystole giving rise to a diamond shape on phonocardiography, but its precise configuration varies widely with the degree of obstruction and other factors. The murmur may be well heard over the carotid arteries but not necessarily so. There may or may not be an accompanying systolic carotid thrill.

The aortic component of the second heart sound will be faint or absent, depending mainly on the mobility of the cusps. If audible it may occur after the pulmonary component, producing reversed splitting with respiration.

Often, but by no means always, there is an accompanying systolic thrill. With significant obstruction, left ventricular hypertrophy will develop and, in due course, left ventricular failure. Reduced ventricular compliance from hypertrophy may be associated with an audible and palpable atrial sound and, with the onset of failure, the murmur becomes quieter and occasionally disappears to reappear after adequate treatment.

Characteristically the murmur has a different quality towards the apex, being of higher pitch and more musical. This fact is one source of confusion in differentiation from the murmur of mitral regurgitation which may of course also be present. The 'ejection' character, with maximum intensity in midsystole is retained.

The difficulty is increased if, as often happens, the heart sounds cannot be heard in the same situation as the murmur, so that precise timing is impossible. It is important to remember that an aortic systolic murmur of no haemodynamic significance is frequently present in the elderly and due to sclerosis of the cusps without a gradient across the valve. If severity of symptoms, or evidence of left ventricular hypertrophy, indicate that surgical treatment may be necessary, it is essential to be certain that obstruction to left ventricular outflow is at valve level.

If an ejection sound is audible or if the valve is calcified there is no difficulty, but in the absence of these signs the alternative possibilities of sub- or more rarely supravalvar obstruction must be considered. Details of differential diagnosis are discussed on page 107.

AORTIC REGURGITATION

The characteristic sign of an aortic regurgitation is a diastolic murmur which begins with the second sound, continues throughout diastole and is of a blowing quality, maximal at the left sternal border.

With severe regurgitation and reduction of ventricular compliance from hypertrophy or left ventricular failure, the diastolic pressure will be raised and the murmur in consequence progressively abbreviated. Frequently there are signs also of aortic stenosis but an aortic systolic murmur from the increased stroke output may be present without a gradient across the valve, especially if the cusps are abnormal.

The severity of regurgitation may be indicated by peripheral signs such as exaggerated, carotid pulsation (Corrigan's sign), a collapsing (water hammer) brachial pulse and by left ventricular enlargement or hypertrophy. However, in the presence of associated aortic stenosis the brachial and carotid pulses are bisferiens in character.

In the absence of corroborative signs it is not possible to differentiate an early diastolic murmur at the left sternal border due to aortic regurgitation from one due to pulmonary regurgitation by auscultation alone.

Aortic regurgitation, like aortic stenosis, is a matter of degree and in clinical practice the whole spectrum of severity is found.

Mild aortic regurgitation is probably the most benign of all acquired valve defects because the left ventricle is well able to compensate for the increase in stroke volume for a life of normal span. However, there is always the risk of infective endocarditis.

When resulting from rheumatic fever the mitral valve is usually, but not always, also affected.

TRICUSPID VALVE DISEASE

Auscultatory signs of rheumatic tricuspid valve disease are often overlooked. This is partly because its presence is not specifically considered in every patient with rheumatic heart disease but also because in most cases there are in addition murmurs from mitral and often aortic valve disease.

Diagnosis is facilitated by initial observation of the jugular venous pulse. Most patients with severe tricuspid stenosis maintain sinus rhythm and an exaggerated and characteristically flicking presystolic wave from atrial systole may be observed, particularly if the patient is reclining at only a few degrees from the horizontal. Initial detection of this sign should lead to the correct interpretation of the presystolic murmur. This murmur is often exceptionally clear, appears to originate close under the stethoscope and increases on inspiration. The y descent of the jugular venous pulse will often be visibly slower than normal and this sign is of course still present in patients with atrial fibrillation.

The mid-diastolic murmur of tricuspid stenosis is usually best heard between the sternum and the apex, does not have the characteristic, rumbling quality of that due to mitral stenosis and, by contrast, it increases with inspiration.

Likewise, in tricuspid regurgitation a pansystolic murmur is often audible in the same region and increases or only becomes audible during deep inspiration. However, if the patient is in right heart failure and the right ventricle is already maximally loaded in expiration there may be no changes on inspiration.

If there is right sided cardiac enlargement with clockwise rotation, as viewed from the apex, the murmur will be loudest at the apex. Occasionally, with extreme mitral stenosis and low blood flow the tricuspid systolic murmur may be the *only* auscultatory sign in a patient with severe mitral stenosis.

In tricuspid regurgitation there will be a systolic wave in the jugular venous pulse followed by a steep y descent, and systolic pulsation of the liver.

Tricuspid regurgitation may result with right ventricular failure from any cause.

COARCTATION OF THE AORTA

The systolic murmur originating at the site of obstruction in the descending aorta is loudest over the spine but usually also audible anteriorly.

There may also be a systolic murmur from a frequently associated, bicuspid aortic valve, from calcific stenosis in such a valve, and sometimes from dilated collateral vessels. With complete occlusion of the aorta there will be no murmur from the area of coarctation but usually loud systolic murmurs from collateral vessels.

With severe narrowing but incomplete obstruction there may be a continuous murmur over the spine and anteriorly the diastolic component may be mistaken for aortic regurgitation.

An aortic diastolic murmur may be present from congenital malformation of the valve or to dilatation of the valve ring secondary to the systemic hypertension. Rarely an apical diastolic murmur is present for which no satisfactory explanation has yet been advanced.

PATENT DUCTUS ARTERIOSUS

The characteristic sign is a continuous murmur which is maximal in late systole and loudest at the upper left sternal border or a little further out. There may or may not be an accompanying thrill.

With a large run-off from aorta to pulmonary artery there may be a somewhat collapsing pulse, an apical diastolic murmur from the increased blood flow across the mitral valve, a prominent hyperkinetic left ventricular impulse and reversed splitting of the second heart sound.

PULMONARY VALVE STENOSIS

The characteristic signs are a harsh systolic murmur and thrill at the upper left sternal border together with an ejection click, maximal on expiration and becoming softer or disappearing on inspiration. With severe stenosis there will be a right ventricular thrust and often an exaggerated *a* wave in the jugular venous pulse and a presystolic gallop rhythm.

Pulmonary stenosis may be associated with a left-to-right shunt or right-to-left shunt at atrial or ventricular level.

'Sometimes the obstruction to right ventricular outflow is at subvalvar level involving the infundibulum of the right ventricle. The differential diagnosis and clinical features of pulmonary stenosis are discussed more fully on page 109.

ATRIAL SEPTAL DEFECT

The characteristic signs are audible splitting of the second heart sound in expiration with fixed splitting during inspiration, and a pulmonary systolic murmur.

With a large flow across the tricuspid valve there will be a corresponding inspiratory tricuspid diastolic murmur and right ventricular lift.

If there is a systolic murmur at the apex, an ostium primum defect with a cleft mitral valve should be suspected.

Anomalous pulmonary venous drainage

When the pulmonary veins drain directly or indirectly into the right atrium, the physical signs are similar to those of an atrial septal defect, but if the atrial septum is intact the second sound will be normally split.

VENTRICULAR SEPTAL DEFECT

The characteristic signs of a ventricular septal defect (VSD) are a pansystolic murmur and thrill maximal at the left sternal border. A thrill is not always present. When there is a large gradient across the defect, that is, when the defect is small and right ventricular (RV) pressure is low, the systolic murmur is long because it extends throughout the period in which pressure in the left ventricle exceeds that in the right. In most cases this would be throughout systole. In some, owing to obstruction to RV outflow at valve or subvalvar level or when the defect is large, producing pulmonary hypertension, the murmur is abbreviated.

With a large shunt there will also be increased blood flow across the mitral valve and consequently a diastolic murmur and/or a third heart sound at the apex.

A reversed (right-to-left) shunt does not itself cause a murmur but a systolic murmur is often present from associated obstruction to RV outflow.

The splitting of the second heart sound may be a little wider than normal. This may be due to shortening of LV systole, due to the double exit for blood, with early closure of the aortic valve and prolongation of RV systole from the increased stroke volume. If there is pulmonary hypertension the pulmonary component will be loud and splitting narrow.

In a very large VSD with RV pressure equal to LV and no associated RV outflow obstruction, as in Eisenmenger's complex, the second sound is single and there may be no systolic murmur at all.

FALLOT'S TETRALOGY

Fallot's tetralogy consists of a large ventricular septal defect, obstruction to right ventricular outflow at infundibular or valve level, dextroposition of the aortic root which lies astride the septal defect, and right ventricular hypertrophy.

The characteristic signs are central cyanosis with clubbing of the fingers and polycythaemia, and a pulmonary systolic murmur. The right to left shunt does not itself produce a murmur. There is no right ventricular lift because of the double exit for blood from the right ventricle.

In contrast to isolated pulmonary stenosis there is no ejection click or presystolic gallop rhythm.

In Fallot's tetralogy the obstruction to RV outflow is most commonly at infundibular level but may occur at valve level or at both. The infundibular stenosis is partly 'fixed' due to a musculofibrous ring but is accompanied by a variable degree of infundibular systolic 'shut-down' due to the hypertrophied muscle of the RV outflow tract obstructing the exit of blood when it contracts. The degree of 'shut down' influences the character of the pulmonary systolic murmur. The greater the 'shut-down' the shorter wil be the murmur. The systolic murmur of Fallot's tetralogy ends with or before A_2 and does not continue through A_2 to P_2 as it may do in pulmonary stenosis with an intact interventricular septum, probably because of the alternative pathway for exit of blood from the right ventricle via the VSD.

The aorta is large and somewhat anterior and usually there is a loud, clear, single second sound due to the aortic component. When the aorta is large, an ejection click of *aortic* valve origin may occasionally be heard in Fallot's tetralogy and is quite commonly heard in pulmonary atresia, which in many ways resembles Fallot's tetralogy but with complete obstruction of the RV outflow instead of just pulmonary stenosis. In pulmonary atresia there is no pulmonary systolic murmur, but often a continuous murmur due to blood flow through greatly dilated bronchial arteries.

CONGENITAL HEART DISEASE IN INFANCY

The diagnosis of congenital heart disease in infancy is often complex and difficult and requires special experience. This subject will not therefore be discussed detail. However, it may be mentioned that both palliative and corrective surgical treatment can be carried out successfully at this age. Consequently, specialist cardiological advice should be sought as early as possible after birth.

In childhood physical signs of congenital heart disease are very similar to those in adults.

Further reading

Craige E 1975 Echocardiography in studies of the genesis of heart sounds and murmurs. In: Yu, Goodwin (eds) Progress in cardiology. Lea and Febiger, Philadelphia

Leatham A 1970 Auscultation of the heart and phonocardiography. Churchill, London

Mckusick V 1958 Cardiovascular sound in health and disease. Williams and Wilkins, Baltimore

Stein P D 1981 A physical and physiological basis for the interpretation of cardiac auscultation. Futura, New York

Index